MW01644942

Dementia Care Confidence

3 STEPS TO TRANSFORM FAMILY CAREGIVING WITH CONFIDENT CARE LEADERSHIP

DR. ANNA THOMAS, MD

Dementia Care Confidence

ISBN Paperback (979-8-9912538-0-2)
ISBN Hardcover (979-8-9912538-1-9)
ISBN EBOOK (979-899125382-6)

First edition 2024

Dedication

This book is dedicated to my parents who taught me the meaning of unconditional love

Preface

Over the past decade, my work as a physician and caregiving coach has allowed me to support thousands of families in their journey with dementia. Each family's story has left a profound mark on me, shaping my understanding and approach to dementia caregiving. Through their experiences and stories, I've learned the true meaning of caregiving, and I hope this book honors all that they've taught me.

To protect the privacy of those I've worked with, all identifiable information and names have been changed, but the essence of their experiences remains in the stories I share. Some of these experiences will take the form of letters introducing each chapter, others as anecdotes and case studies throughout the book.

This book is intended to be a practical guide designed to equip you with the knowledge and tools needed to lead with compassion and confidence in the face of dementia care. As you read through the pages, I invite you to reflect on your journey and embrace the principles of care leadership.

Finally, I wish to take a moment to express my deepest gratitude to my beloved husband, Cyril Thomas, and my children, Sara and George. Their unwavering support, endless love, and patience have been my constant source of strength.

With gratitude,

Dr. Anna Thomas

Contents

INTRODUCTION 1

STEP 1: LEAD YOURSELF 11

1. Are You a Care Leader? 13
2. Your Caregiving Style 17
3. Growth Mindset & Limiting Beliefs 27
4. Self-Care is a Leadership Requirement 39

STEP 2: LEAD THE CARE PARTNERSHIP 53

5. Dementia & the Care Partnership 55
6. Your Care Partner's Needs & Abilities 61
7. Relationship Mindset & Limiting Beliefs in Care Partnerships 73
8. Communication Changes in Dementia 83

STEP 3: LEAD THE CARE TEAM 99

9. Why You Need a Team 101
10. Building Your Team 105
11. Leader's Mindset & Limiting Beliefs 117
12. Team Coordination & Management 125

ENSURING YOUR LONG TERM SUCCESS 137

INTRODUCTION

There are only four kinds of people
in the world.
Those who have been caregivers.
Those who are currently caregivers.
Those who will be caregivers, and
Those who will need a caregiver

Rosalyn Carter

INTRODUCTION

Dear Dr. Thomas,

I am writing because I desperately need advice on a very difficult issue with my mother's care. I brought her home with me after her last hospital stay because she can't live alone anymore.

The problem is that I can't find anyone reliable to help me. My mom doesn't adapt well to new people, and the agency I hired keeps sending new people every day. On top of that, the agency aides are often late, and when they do arrive, they spend all their time on their cellphones.

I'm trying to do all of this while also working from home. My boss has been supportive so far, but I don't know how long that will last. At some point, I have to get my work done too, and there is a push for us to come back to the office in person soon.

What do I do?

Julie

Dementia is a common and devastating medical problem impacting millions of people worldwide. Dementia itself isn't a single diagnosis but a term that describes a collection of different ones ranging from Alzheimer's disease to Lewy Body dementia, vascular dementia, and more. While the causes of each of these diseases can vary, ultimately they all lead to a similar path and share similar features, like difficulty with learning and retaining new memories, problem-solving, language issues, and difficulty functioning independently. According to Alzheimer's Disease International and the World Health Organization, more than ten million people are diagnosed with dementia every year.[12] This staggering number is only expected to increase.

The challenge with dementia is that it's a progressive condition with no known cure. Over time, as dementia advances, the person with dementia needs more help managing their day-to-day needs and eventually becomes completely dependent on others. This growing need for care is typically met by informal family caregivers—most often women in their forties to sixties, providing hundreds of hours of unpaid care to a loved one with dementia, all while trying to work and manage their own personal lives and families as well. The value of the work these caregivers provide for the aging population is astronomical—more than $200 billion in the US alone, according to a study published by the Alzheimer's Association in 2015.[3]

Imagine a caregiver like Susan, who starts her day at five a.m. to prepare breakfast for her family, then spends hours assisting her mother with basic needs like bathing and dressing. By noon, she's exhausted but still has to manage household chores, her job, and her children's needs. By the time she goes to bed, she's barely had a moment to breathe, let alone care for herself.

The last four years have been especially difficult for caregivers because of the COVID pandemic. Reliable resources for these caregivers were scarce to begin with, and many home care agencies struggled to provide adequate staffing even for the families able to pay the high cost of private services. Most family support groups were closed during the pandemic, and online forums had more questions than answers. Information on the internet continues to be fragmented and confusing, and healthcare providers primarily focus on prescriptions, without much regard for the struggles of the caregivers who had to ensure those medications were actually taken.

Elaine's story illustrates the challenges faced by many caregivers. She discovered the severity of her dad's cognitive decline after a year of pandemic-induced isolation. Her once vibrant, strong, and reliable dad had become an anxious shell of his former self. He had started hoarding, and stacks of papers, clothing, and household trash filled his living spaces.

Elaine did her best to step up. She flew into town every weekend to sort through the mess, settle overdue bills, and convince her father to move to her home. However, paranoia made him push her away, accusing her of stealing and throwing away his belongings. He refused to let her join him at his medical appointments and insisted he could drive safely. Soon, Elaine was fielding calls from her siblings who had refused to help meaningfully, now complaining that she was upsetting the status quo by pointing out their father's decline. She realized there was no one coming to her rescue. There was no help, just her.

Many caregivers have to deal with chronic stress, anxiety, and depression associated with caregiving responsibilities. The constant worry about their loved one's well-being, coupled with the lack of support, can be crushing. Relationships with family and friends often become strained. Marital stress, conflicts with siblings over caregiving responsibilities, and a lack of understanding from friends add to the caregiver's burden.

If you are reading this book, chances are you've faced similar challenges like Julie, Susan, and Elaine. Perhaps you too have struggled to figure out a plan to care for your loved one, sought out support groups but kept running into walls, or found yourself handling these tasks all by yourself, with little support from your family. You may have felt alone and overwhelmed and wondered, *"How do I get through this? Is it even possible?"*

I was first introduced to dementia when I was in 9th grade when we went to visit my grandmother in India. I remember feeling shocked when my grandmother asked me who I was, whether I was married, and why I was staying with them. Shouldn't I be going home to my own house by now? Won't my children be waiting for me? She had forgotten who I was and that I was still a child.

In later years, I saw the horrific confusion, delusions, and memory changes that she had to go through. I also saw the challenges my parents faced as they stepped in to care for her, trying to balance her care needs with those of my brother and I as we entered our college years. Struggling with long-distance caregiving, my father quit his job, moved back to India, and spent a year taking care of his mother in her last year of life.

In many ways, my family's experiences with aging and dementia care shaped my path to where I am today, leading me to become a physician specializing in internal medicine (medical care for adults) and hospice and palliative care (medical care for those at or near the end stages of life). In the past decade, working as a board-certified physician, I've had the privilege of helping thousands of patients with advanced dementia diagnoses.

The longer I've worked as a physician, the more I've come to understand that the caregiver is essential to the dementia care puzzle. This caregiver, who might be a spouse, wife, sister, or even just a good friend who's taken it upon themselves to step in, is the key factor to the success of any medical options I might offer as a doctor. Without the caregiver, there can be no plan or no medical intervention.

I've also witnessed first-hand that there is far too little support for caregivers, who struggle under the weight of the task. I've witnessed this not only in my professional role but also in my family. I've learned that most caregivers start their journey with dementia care overwhelmed by disorganized information, lacking clear guidance, and silently fearing how to handle the emotional and practical challenges that this caregiving responsibility brings.

In today's world, caregiving is unsustainable without proper support. The caregivers I've seen struggle most, however, have been the ones who saw their role simply as caregivers, literally just "givers of care." They gave and gave and gave some more, following all the best advice, but they couldn't thrive despite it.

> *When you're caring for someone with dementia, you will lose yourself in the giving if you're not careful.*

If you're a caregiver of a loved one with dementia, I caution you to stop for a moment and reread this: *you will lose yourself if you don't approach caregiving differently.* As the disease progresses and changes, your loved one needs more and more from you; not just physical and practical needs, but also emotional support, decision-making, and more.

The women I saw who most successfully handled and adapted to the increasing demands didn't see themselves simply as givers of care. They saw themselves as something more, as care *leaders*. They recognized that what they had been called to do was not just to follow but, over time, take the reins and lead. When you view your role from the lens of a leadership perspective rather than of a simple giver of care, everything changes.

With leadership skills, caregivers can learn how to balance their needs and those of their loved ones. They learn to think strategically, looking at the big picture. They start to see their energy and time as a finite and precious resource that needs to be allocated for leading and they learn to create a team to help them carry out the day-to-day tasks that dementia care demands. Care leaders also recognize that caring for someone with dementia is unique from all other care relationships because it's a partnership between you and the person you love, a person whose needs and abilities change every day.

Let me share a few examples:

- Maryann, a coaching client of mine, had been caring for her husband with early-onset Alzheimer's dementia for the past two years. They have no children and no family nearby to help her. After working with me, she understood that her first responsibility as a leader was to develop and nurture herself, learn how to communicate with her husband and create a support team for herself.

- Betty, another client, had never viewed herself as a leader. Her highly intelligent, highly successful husband had always been the decision-maker in the house until he was diagnosed with vascular dementia. Through our program, Betty learned to assess the situation thoroughly, and confidently step into a leadership role she'd never had to hold before.

What each coaching client learned can be summarized in this simple concept: *You are more than just a caregiver; you are a Care Leader*. Being a care leader requires a different mindset, one of foresight, decision-making, and self-care. With the right guidance, I'm confident that every caregiver, including you, can rise to the challenge.

Through my company, LifeCare LeadHership, my mission is to empower women caregivers like you in your journey to becoming a Care Leader. In this book, I've distilled the essence of my coaching program with the hope that I can spread my mission to more women who need this support.

This book is for you if you're a woman who finds herself in the role of caregiver for a loved one with dementia, whether you stepped into this role willingly or were thrust into it unexpectedly. It's for you if you feel overwhelmed by the responsibilities of caregiving and the unique challenges of caring for someone with dementia. It's for you, my friend, who feels alone and unseen in your caregiving struggle.

I see you.

Whether you feel overwhelmed by caregiving responsibilities or simply desire to enhance your caregiving skills and abilities, this book will be your companion on the journey.

The Confident Care Leader Framework

The Confident Care Leader Framework is the cornerstone of this book. It's designed to empower you to become a confident and compassionate care leader capable of meeting the unique challenges of dementia care head-on. It consists of three fundamental steps, detailed below.

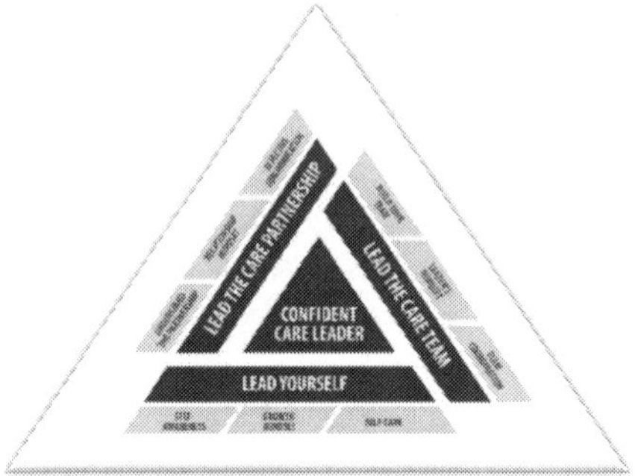

Figure 1: Confident Care Leader Framework

Step 1: Lead Yourself

Caregiving begins with self-leadership. You can't lead anyone until you can first lead yourself well. Through this fundamental stage, you will gain greater self-awareness of your unique caregiving strengths and style, and identify areas for personal growth.

Taking on a caregiving role requires developing a growth mindset and overcoming limiting beliefs that prevent you from accepting change, which we will explore in detail. However, the most essential skill you must develop may be surprising, as it's the most overlooked and dismissed– the ability to prioritize self-care. If you don't do this, you will burn out quickly.

Step 2: Lead the Care Partnership

Effective care leadership hinges on having a solid bond with the person who has dementia. To use a business analogy, your loved one is the CEO *and* the only client of the "company" known as their life. The company's primary purpose is to ensure the client's health, safety, and well-being. So, what's your role? You are the Chief Operating Officer (the COO) of this person's life, ensuring everything runs smoothly. To do that, you need to know exactly what 's going on, so you can create a plan to step in where needed.

In this stage, we'll develop a thorough understanding of dementia and how to get a good assessment of your loved one's needs. After building our awareness of the care partnership and your loved one's condition, we'll overcome the limiting beliefs that affect the relationship mindset. Finally, we'll learn how to communicate and connect with our loved ones.

Step 3: Lead the Care Team

The final step is moving from being a solo caregiver to leading a team of other caregivers. Dementia caregiving requires many different types of skill sets; one person can't easily do all these tasks while still balancing their own life. In this section, we'll first identify how much and what type of help you need, and then discover how to overcome any limiting beliefs about having a team that may be holding you back. In addition, you'll develop leadership skills for communicating with and managing your team to advocate for the very best care for your loved one.

Throughout this book, you'll find exercises, insights, and real-life examples to deepen your understanding and develop your skills as a care leader. Use these resources to nurture your well-being, strengthen your relationship with your loved one with dementia, and effectively lead your care team. You will also find additional resources in this book's online portal, my gift to you, which you can access here:

Access Additional Resources in Your Book Portal:

www.lifecareleadhership.com/dcc

What If I Don’t Want to Be a Caregiver?

Many women who are in caregiving roles didn't come to this role willingly. I know that while I use the words "loved one with dementia" throughout the book to indicate that the person you care for is likely a person you’re close to, for some of you "love" may not be exactly the words you would choose to describe your relationship. You might be feeling stuck or forced into a role you never would’ve chosen for yourself.

While the promise of this book is that if you develop your caregiving and leadership skills with my framework—first for yourself and your care partnership, and then your team—you will transform your caregiving, it doesn’t promise to make you *want* to be a care leader or a caregiver.

I can’t make you want to do the job and take on the responsibilities, and I can’t change your family circumstances, but I still believe that in these pages you’ll find tools to make the work a little bit easier for you. If you go through the book, you’ll find resources to help you create support for yourself and determine the right path forward for you. The more open and honest you are about yourself in the process, the greater the change that you will experience in your life and your caregiving.

Remember, you're not alone on this journey. If you're ready to start, I'll see you in Chapter 1.

Self-Reflection Questions

Before moving on, please complete the quick self-assessment quiz on the next page. I've included the same assessment at the end of the book so that you can look back later and see how much you've grown.

Care Leader Self-Assessment:

Instructions: Rate your confidence level for each statement on a scale from 1 to 10, where 1 = Not Confident and 10 = Very Confident.

1. ________My confidence in understanding and utilizing my unique skills as a care leader.
2. ________My confidence in creating and maintaining a wellness plan for my own well-being.
3. ________My confidence in accurately assessing and understanding the needs of my loved one.
4. ________My confidence in communicating with my loved one to ensure their needs and preferences are met.
5. ________My confidence in identifying the right people to include in my care team.
6. ________My confidence in creating a care plan that enables all team members to work together effectively

1. Alzheimer's Disease International. "World Alzheimer Report 2020: Design, Dignity, Dementia: Dementia-Related Design and the Built Environment." Alzheimer's Disease International, 2020. Available at: https://www.alzint.org/resource/world-alzheimer-report-2020/.

2. World Health Organization. "Dementia: A Public Health Priority." World Health Organization, 2019. Available at: https://www.who.int/news-room/fact-sheets/detail/dementia.

3. Alzheimer's Association. "2015 Alzheimer's Disease Facts and Figures." Alzheimer's Association, 2015. Available at: https://www.alz.org/facts/.

STEP 1: LEAD YOURSELF

In order to grow yourself,
you must know yourself.

John C. Maxwell

One

Are You a Care Leader?

Dear Dr. Thomas,

I went to visit my mom recently and it broke my heart to see her overwhelmed and struggling.

My mom is an elegant and put-together woman, but her house was a complete mess for the first time in my memory. There were papers everywhere and the kitchen counters were stacked with unwashed dishes. It was clear she had stopped doing her laundry a while ago and needed a lot of help.

Standing in her living room, seeing her anxious and worried, I knew I had to step in and help, but I didn't even know where to start.

Honestly, I'm not even sure if I'm the right one to take this on. Can I handle this?

Amy

What Does It Mean to Be a Care Leader?

Many women who are caregivers for loved ones with dementia cannot picture themselves as a leader. Like Amy, they may doubt their capabilities or authority and wonder if they're even up to the task. You aren't alone in thinking these thoughts but whether you realize it or not, you're *already* a leader and can become an even better one, starting today.

Let me start by defining leadership. When most people think about leadership and leaders, they tend to imagine someone who speaks loudly, gives orders, and makes quick decisions. Movies and TV shows often portray leaders as angry, loud men who love to take charge of everything, so if that's what came to your mind, I'm not surprised. It's hard to see yourself as a leader if you don't fit that mold, but the good news is that there are many different types of leaders and leadership styles. In my experience, care leaders can be the quietest person in the room.

Authentic leadership is about having a big-picture plan, guiding the way forward, and empowering everyone in the team. It's less about shouting orders and more about finding ways to make the team succeed. Care leaders understand and embody authentic leadership because they're focused on the person they love with dementia, and work with their small team to provide the best care possible. They are flexible and adaptable, and rely highly on their skills in emotional intelligence (for example, being sensitive to others' feelings) and resilience (staying strong when things get tough). It's a demanding role but also incredibly fulfilling.

Suzanne is a perfect example of a caregiver who transformed her role by embracing leadership. When her husband John started to experience memory concerns, Suzanne was the first to notice. She realized that John was deferring more and more to her judgment over time. Simple decisions were now overwhelming him, such as where to go out to eat and what to get from the grocery store. Then, he started to forget the steps and sequences of activities. She would walk into their bedroom in the morning to find him half-dressed and getting back into bed. She learned that she needed to be more proactive and guide him through the steps of the day.

With support, she learned how to guide her husband and lead their care partnership effectively. It took a lot of time and effort to change some of her old perspectives on who did what in their relationship; but because of the work she did, she grew confident in her skills and ability.

However, one of the first changes Suzanne had to make to embrace this new role was understanding what it means to be a care leader. This kind of powerful leadership centers on the relationship between her and her loved one, emphasizing respect and trust rather than formal titles.

Understanding Self Leadership

Growth is essential for caregivers like you to fulfill your role with confidence and effectiveness. The good news is that leadership skills are learnable!

In this section of the book, you'll discover the foundational elements essential for your growth as a care leader. It all begins with self-leadership—taking charge of your own development and well-being to care for your loved one with dementia effectively.

Let's start by understanding the concept of self-leadership. It's about recognizing that before you can effectively guide someone else, you must have a deep understanding of yourself. This involves self-awareness, or knowing your strengths, weaknesses, values, and motivations. Self-awareness is a powerful tool that allows you to recognize how you respond under stress, what triggers your emotions, and where you need support. By knowing yourself, you can better manage your reactions and make informed decisions in caregiving situations.

Developing a positive mindset and attitude is key in caregiving. It means seeing challenges as opportunities for growth and learning rather than obstacles. Understand that setbacks are part of the journey, and each challenge you overcome strengthens your ability to care for your loved one.

Effective caregiving also requires cultivating various skills, from managing medications to providing emotional support. Continuously improving your skills will increase your confidence and competence as a caregiver.

By embracing self-leadership, you empower yourself to become a more effective and resilient caregiver. This foundational step is crucial for crossing the complexities of dementia care with confidence and compassion. As you lead yourself, you set the stage for leading your loved one through their journey with dementia, ensuring that both of you can thrive despite the challenges.

In the first part of this section, I'll guide you through a self-assessment to build your self-awareness. This will help you identify your current strengths and areas where you can further develop your skills. Understanding your starting point is essential for targeted growth and improvement.

Next, we 'll discover the beliefs holding you back from effective leadership, and how your perspective and approach can profoundly impact how you care for your loved one.

Lastly, we'll focus on the critical skill of self-care for caregivers. By the end of this chapter, you will have practical strategies and insights to help you prioritize your well-being while caring for your loved one. Remember, taking care of yourself isn't a luxury, it's a necessity for providing the best care.

Like many caregivers, Amy and Suzanne faced doubts about their ability to take on the role of care leader. However, they discovered their innate leadership potential through learning and self-reflection and confidently embraced their responsibilities.

By the end of this section, armed with a solid foundation in self-leadership and practical tools for caregiving, you'll be empowered to lead with confidence and compassion as well. Just as Suzanne and Amy transformed their caregiving approach, you too can conquer the challenges of dementia care with confidence!

Self-Reflection Questions

1. How do you currently see your role for your loved one with dementia?

2. Do you believe you are a leader?

Two

Your Caregiving Style

Dear Dr. Thomas,

My sister Melissa and I care for our elderly parents, who live in a nearby assisted living facility. Melissa visits our parents daily and does a lot of hands-on stuff like taking them to the bathroom or helping Mom shower on the weekends.

My approach is quite different. I don't really want to do baths or toileting—we are paying a lot of money for the facility, and I feel we can rely on them for these kinds of small daily actions. I instead make it a point to meet regularly with the supervisors and coordinate with all the doctors.

Would you still consider me a caregiver or more of a coordinator for my parents' care? Is there a different term for what I do?

Thank You,

Melanie

What is the "Best" Caregiving Style?

In the last chapter, we explored what it means to be a care leader, but a common question I get is what it means to be a good caregiver. Most people assume that all caregiving is hands-on, meaning you handle tasks like toileting, bathing, and dressing the individual when they can no longer do it themselves. The reality is that there are many different needs for a loved one with dementia, and just as many ways to meet those needs.

Understanding your unique caregiving style helps you become a stronger leader. The more self-aware you are, the more you know your unique strengths, areas where caregiving is easy for you, and areas where you need to supplement with the help of other team members. What's most important to remember is that there's no single "best" style, just whatever works best for you and your family. Some caregivers, like Melissa, thrive in the hands-on aspects of care, whereas others, like Melanie, prefer to focus on organization and coordination. Both approaches are needed, and both sisters should be considered care leaders.

The DISC Model & Your Caregiving Style

As part of my Confident Care Leader Program, I encourage my coaching clients to really take the time to understand their unique personalities using the DISC model. It's a well-established methodology for helping people better understand themselves through their strengths, weaknesses, areas for growth, and communication ability. It was initially developed in 1928 by William Moulton Marston, as a tool for behavioral theory, but over the past century, it's been used in many industries, including corporate environments, healthcare, and government sectors.

The DISC model is based on the idea that there are four main personality styles: Dominant (D), Influence (I), Steadiness (S), and Conscientiousness (C). Each style has its own unique characteristics and features. However, it's important to know that every person can be a blend of these styles, combining traits such as assertiveness or meticulousness to create a unique care leader. Let's discover how these four main styles apply to caregiving.

Dominant (D) Style Caregiver: Dominant-style caregivers are excellent at organizing, planning, and executing tasks. For instance, Melanie, whom we read about at the start of this chapter, is a primary D-style care leader. She creates a detailed weekly schedule for her mother with dementia, coordinates medical appointments, and advocates for her parents with the assisted living supervisors when needed. Melanie, like other D-style individuals, tends to be decisive and quick to take action.

Influence (I) Style Caregiver: Bringing enthusiasm and positivity, influence-style caregivers motivate and support their loved ones emotionally. Emma, a coaching client of mine, for example, always greets her father, who is in the early stages of dementia, with a smile and encouraging words. She's excellent at planning engaging activities like painting and gardening, consistently uplifting his spirits. Emma's optimistic outlook fosters engagement and a sense of love and support for her loved one.

Steadiness (S) Style Caregiver: Nurturing and compassionate, steadiness-style caregivers prioritize emotional and physical comfort. Melissa, a primary S-style caregiver, spends quality time with her mother and provides hands-on assistance. She assists with daily tasks like dressing and bathing and offers reassurance and warmth through her gentle demeanor. Melissa's presence provides security and peace, an excellent skill set for any caregiver.

Conscientiousness (C) Style Caregiver: Conscientious-style caregivers focus on thorough analysis and problem-solving. Sarah, another coaching client, meticulously tracks her husband's symptoms and medication effects, documenting changes in behavior or health precisely. She researches the latest dementia treatments and discusses options with healthcare providers to ensure the best care plan.

It's essential to remember that each caregiving style brings unique strengths and contributions to the caregiving journey. Recognizing and embracing your primary style is important. The more you know about yourself, the more you can leverage your strengths and address areas for growth so that you can become an even better care leader.

If you're unsure about your caregiving style, take the following quick five-question quiz to gain insights into your natural tendencies and preferences when providing care.

Exercise: Your Caregiving Style Quiz

Instructions: For each question, select the answer that best describes how you typically behave or feel in caregiving situations.

1. When faced with a caregiving task, what is your initial reaction?

(A) Take charge and start organizing a plan of action.
(B) Uplift the person needing care, providing emotional support.
(C) Listening and understanding their needs before acting.
(D) Analyze the situation thoroughly before deciding.

2. How do you prefer to communicate with the person you're caring for?

(A) Directly and assertively, providing clear instructions.
(B) Positively and cheerfully, offering words of encouragement.
(C) Empathetically and patiently, listening to their concerns.
(D) Logically presenting information in a systematic manner.

3. What motivates you the most in your caregiving role

(A) Achieving tangible results and accomplishing tasks efficiently.
(B) Seeing the person you care for happy and uplifted.
(C) Building emotional connections and providing comfort.
(D) Solving problems and finding practical solutions to challenges.

4. When faced with a difficult decision in caregiving, what guides your choice

(A) What will lead to the most effective and efficient outcome.
(B) What will bring the most joy to the person in need.
(C) What aligns with their emotional well-being and comfort.
(D) What is the most rational and logical decision

5. How do you feel most fulfilled in your caregiving role?

(A) When tasks are completed successfully, and in order.

(B) When you see the person you care for smiling & supported.

(C) When you know you've provided comfort and stability.

(D) When you've solved problems and overcome challenges.

Scoring & Interpretation: Your highest score determines your primary caregiving style.

For each (a) answer: 1 point for Dominant

For each (b) answer: 1 point for Influence

For each (c) answer: 1 point for Steadiness

For each (d) answer: 1 point for Conscientiousness

What Can You Learn About Yourself When You Know Your Style?

Understanding your caregiving style offers deep insights into your strengths and areas for growth. It helps you grasp how you naturally interact with your loved one and guides you in enhancing your effectiveness as a care leader.

Book Portal Resource Alert!

Want a Full Assessment & Comprehensive Report?

Visit your book portal at www.lifecareleadhership.com/dcc

If you're a dominant style caregiver, your strengths lie in being organized and decisive. You excel at planning and ensuring that daily routines and medical needs are met efficiently. Your quick decision-making helps solve problems promptly. However, you may tend to be inflexible at times and find it challenging to adjust to unexpected changes. Recognizing these tendencies can help you become more adaptable and patient, which are valuable traits in caregiving.

Like a cheerleader, if you're an influence-style caregiver you bring a hopeful and uplifting attitude that significantly boosts your loved one's spirits. You excel at encouraging participation in activities that keep them engaged. However, your optimism might sometimes lead you to overlook serious issues, and maintaining a constantly positive attitude can be emotionally draining. Balancing optimism with a realistic outlook and taking time for self-care is essential to prevent burnout in this emotionally demanding role.

If you're a steadiness-style caregiver, you're deeply compassionate, providing comfort and emotional support with patience and kindness. You prioritize creating a nurturing environment. However, your nurturing nature may occasionally lead to overprotectiveness, limiting your loved one's independence. You can grow by encouraging their independence and remembering to care for yourself. This balance helps maintain your well-being and prevents caregiver fatigue.

Like an analyst, if you're a conscientiousness-style caregiver you are detail-oriented and excel at problem-solving. You carefully monitor symptoms and research treatments to ensure informed care decisions. However, focusing too much on details can sometimes lead to overthinking and emotional distance. Finding a balance between analytical thinking and emotional connection is key to enhancing the caregiving relationship and making timely decisions.

> Now, take a moment to think about your own caregiving style after reading this. Do you see yourself as more of a dominant-style, an influence-style, a steadiness-style, or a conscientiousness-style caregiver?

In my previous caregiving roles, as both a mother and a daughter, I fell into the steadiness and conscientiousness categories. While I excelled in providing emotional support and maintaining a nurturing environment, I also valued organization and attention to detail. However, I realized that I needed to strengthen my skills from other categories to become a more effective caregiver. I worked on making quicker decisions and bringing positivity into my interactions, incorporating elements of the dominant and influence styles.

Identifying Areas for Self-Growth

Discovering and nurturing your leadership skills is pivotal when on the path to becoming an effective care leader. As a caregiver growing into a care leader, the four key areas that are essential to develop over time include:

Knowledge & Practical Skills: Caring for someone with a complex medical illness requires you to deepen your knowledge and understanding of their illness, how it's treated, and what to expect over time. Practical skills include how to provide hands-on care, how to change or bathe someone who is bedbound, or how to make sure medications are given correctly. Of these four areas, this one may feel like the biggest hurdle but these skills are actually the easiest ones to acquire.

> *Self-Reflection: On a scale of 1 (low) to 5 (high), rate how well you understand what is going on with your loved one's medical condition and how comfortable you feel with the practical skills required for day-to-day management.*

Communication & Intrapersonal Skills: Mere knowledge isn't enough; for care leaders to be effective, they need to know how to convey this information clearly, respectfully, and with empathy. These "soft" skills are often overlooked but are so important in both caregiving and managing a team.

> *Self-Reflection: Rate your current level of communication and intrapersonal skills in caregiving from 1 to 5.*

Organizational & Time Management Skills: As a care leader, managing various responsibilities efficiently is crucial for smoothly operating caregiving tasks. This includes scheduling appointments, managing medications, coordinating care plans, and maintaining a safe and comfortable environment. Solid organizational skills help prevent oversights, reduce stress, and provide structure, allowing you to focus more on meaningful interactions and quality care.

Self-Reflection: How well do you manage the day-to-day tasks of caregiving? Rate your organizational skills on a scale of 1 to 5.

Problem-Solving & Strategic Planning Skills: Challenges are inevitable in caregiving, and developing strong problem-solving abilities are essential. Care leaders must assess each situation calmly and rationally, identify potential solutions, and decide on a strategic plan that addresses the unique needs and preferences of those they care for.

Self-Reflection: On a scale of 1 to 5, rate your current problem-solving and strategic planning abilities in caregiving.

This book covers a lot of ground to help you grow in the four areas above, but I would also love to share a couple of my favorite resources with you.

Some of My Favorite Recommendations

1. *The 36-Hour Day: A Family Guide to Caring for People Who Have Alzheimer's Disease, Related Dementias, and Memory Loss*, by Nancy L. Mace and Peter V. Rabins (Hopkins Press, 2021)

2. *Positive Approach to Care Training videos,* by Teepa Snows , available on YouTube: https://www.youtube.com/@teepasnowvideos

3. *Crucial Conversations: Tools for Talking When Stakes Are High,* by Kerry Patterson, Joseph Grenny, Ron McMillan, and Al Switzler (McGraw-Hill, 2002)

4. *Everyone Communicates, Few Connect: What the Most Effective People Do Differently,* by John C Maxwell (HarperCollins Leadership, 2010)

5. *First Things First*, by Stephen Covey (Franklin Covey Co., 1996)

Remember, nurturing ongoing growth and development is essential for caregivers and leaders. By investing in yourself through these resources, you can enhance your skills, gain confidence, and become a more effective and compassionate caregiver. Each step you take in developing these skills improves your caregiving abilities and strengthens the bond and trust between you and those you care for.

Self-Reflection Questions

1. What have you learned about yourself and your caregiving style that was new or unexpected?
2. Of the four areas of growth mentioned in this chapter, which will you focus on first?

Three

Growth Mindset & Limiting Beliefs

Dear Dr. Thomas,

I recently brought my father, who has Parkinson's dementia, home to stay with me.

It's been quite a challenge—I've got all this medical equipment to manage, new meds to keep track of, and a pretty complicated routine to follow. Honestly, I'm feeling a bit overwhelmed. I keep questioning whether I'm really up for this.

You see, I made a promise to my dad that I'd do everything possible to keep him out of a nursing home. But now that he's here, I'm not sure I have all the skills and know-how to handle everything he needs.

It's a lot to take on. Do you think I made a mistake bringing him home with me?

Best regards,

Amanda

New Roles, New Changes

In the introduction to this section, I shared with you the concept of self-leadership and the fact that all caregivers are leaders. You may have accepted the fact that you're a leader, after all, you do have great responsibility, but do you feel like one?

In our minds, transitioning from a mere giver of care to one leading the team isn't a simple step. For some of us, it can feel like a huge step, and it may feel like a step filled with doubt and self-sabotage. We may actively try to talk ourselves out of taking on this role or, worse, talk ourselves down about our own abilities and strengths. Have you ever felt this way?

Perhaps you've had moments when you felt overwhelmed by the daily challenges, questioning whether you're truly capable of managing everything. Maybe you've compared yourself to others, feeling like you're falling short or don't have what it takes to lead effectively. These feelings are common, and it's natural to experience uncertainty and self-doubt, especially when faced with the immense responsibility of caregiving. You're not alone in these thoughts, and it's important to acknowledge them as a part of your journey.

I urge you to realize that we all carry around an inner critic. This inner critic is ready to pounce on our dreams and aspirations with the misguided goal of keeping us safe. The critic uses **limiting beliefs**, which are negative beliefs we have about ourselves and the world, against us to restrict us.

Why is this important? Our beliefs shape our mindset, which is how we view the world and our abilities, and influence our self-worth and self-confidence. In caregiving, these negative beliefs might manifest as doubts about our capacity to manage complex situations, fears of making wrong decisions, or feelings of inadequacy in providing the best care.

Many people who are new to leadership and caregiving roles hold onto these limiting beliefs and then internalize them to mean something about us. Our capacity (or perceived lack of capacity) to manage complex situations for our loved ones becomes internalized and generalized to our capacity to manage complex situations in all settings.

Do you see how this can erode your self-worth and self-confidence?

I encourage you to ignore the inner critic holding you back and to adopt what's known as a **growth mindset**, which is the self-belief that you can always change, grow, and become a better leader, from today until the end of your life. No one is born knowing how to be a caregiver; all of us must learn and develop these skills, and so can you.

Shifting your perspective can help you overcome these limiting beliefs. By recognizing and challenging these thoughts, you can transform your mindset (how you think about things) and your approach to caregiving. This shift involves acknowledging your skills and strengths and being open to learning and growth.

Common limiting beliefs that caregivers often hold include:

- "I'm not qualified to manage this."
- "I need to do everything perfectly."
- "I have to do everything myself."

Let's study how to reframe these three limiting beliefs next.

Perspective Shift#1: "I'm Not Qualified to Manage This" to… "I have the Skills & Knowledge I Need, *AND* I'm Open to Learning More."

Transitioning into a caregiving role often stirs up significant feelings of self-doubt and uncertainty. For many new dementia caregivers like Amanda, the sudden responsibility of managing medication changes, handling medical equipment, and juggling new routines can feel overwhelming. Even caregivers who have prior nursing experience can struggle with all the care needs of a person with dementia, it's common to start to question your abilities and qualifications when you're getting started.

Initially, Amanda wrestled with guilt and hesitation, questioning her capabilities to navigate the complexities of dementia care. However, as she continued to care for her father, she started to gain confidence in her abilities. She learned through practical experience and took incremental steps that shifted her mindset from "I'm not qualified" to "I have the skills and knowledge I need, *and* I'm open to learning more."

Amanda began by researching her father's condition and implementing small, manageable routines that improved their daily life. Celebrating small victories, like establishing a consistent schedule that eased her father's anxiety, boosted her confidence. Day by day, she witnessed the positive impact of her efforts on her father's well-being, reinforcing her belief in her capabilities.

Through her journey, Amanda discovered that she had the capacity but also qualifications to be her father's care leader. She realized that she could leverage skills that she had developed in other areas of her life and apply them to her caregiving role. She grew into the role gracefully and confidently, finding strength in her experiences.

Have you also struggled with self-doubt? If so, the following exercise will help you reframe this belief.

Exercise: Recognizing Your Caregiving Skills

1. **Make a List:** Set a timer for two minutes. During these two minutes, jot down all the caregiving tasks you've handled today. Include everything from waking your loved one to preparing meals, managing medications, providing companionship and support, and more
2. **Reflect**: After writing, reflect on each task and recognize the effort and skill required. Don't underestimate the importance of even the most minor actions in caregiving.
3. **Acknowledge Your Abilities**: Take a moment to review your list. Appreciate all that you do and recognize the impact of your caregiving efforts. This exercise is a powerful reminder of the many ways you're already skilled and capable in your caregiving role.

Chances are, you'll fill that paper with numerous tasks you manage effortlessly every day. that you hadn't even been thinking about. It's important to recognize and appreciate these abilities. Perhaps there are tasks you're unsure about, like managing medical equipment or changing wound dressings. Remember, you can learn these skills or even choose to delegate them to somebody else.

Understanding your capabilities and being open to learning new skills or seeking assistance is the first step in reframing this limiting belief. Remember: You're capable of more than you realize!

Perspective Shift# 2: "I Need to Do Everything Perfectly" to... "I Need to Do Things Well, but it Doesn't Have to Be Perfect."

The secret to feeling fulfilled is being aware that you're doing a decent job, even when you don't feel that way. Unfortunately, many caregivers struggle with this feeling, always aiming for perfection. Let's look at Donna's story, for example.

> *Donna's Challenge*: Donna faced a daunting caregiving situation. Her mother's advanced dementia and blindness made communication and daily care exceptionally challenging. Donna took immense pride in her responsibility as her mother's caregiver. She was meticulous in every detail, ensuring her mother received the best care possible. Donna didn't trust anyone else to handle her mother's needs, believing she alone understood her mom's routines and preferences.
>
> However, one incident shattered Donna's confidence. One day, despite her vigilant care, her mother attempted to rise from a chair unassisted and fell, breaking her wrist in the process. Donna was devastated. She blamed herself for not foreseeing the fall and preventing it. This moment shook her deeply, making her question every decision she had ever made as a caregiver. She felt she had failed in her most important role—to keep her mother safe and comfortable.

> The fall triggered a wave of self-doubt for Donna. She scrutinized her approach, wondering if she could've done more to prevent such incidents. Ultimately, she realized there wasn't anything more she could've done short of wrapping her mom in bubble wrap. The event forced her to confront the harsh reality that accidents could still happen even under her cautious care.

In caregiving, striving for perfection can often lead to undue stress and unrealistic expectations. It's important to recognize and set realistic standards that prioritize safety while acknowledging the challenges of caring for someone with dementia. A helpful approach to reframing limiting beliefs around perfectionism is to rewrite our goals or standards using the good/better/best framework.

How does this framework work? Our goal in caregiving is to aim for an acceptable standard, "good," consistently, with some days achieving "better" and occasionally reaching "best." This balanced approach ensures we maintain realistic expectations and prioritize our loved one's well-being and ours as well.

Try the Good/Better/Best framework using the exercise below.

Exercise: Applying Good/Better/Best

1. **Get Prepared:** Grab a fresh piece of paper and prepare to journal for at least ten to twenty minutes on this topic.
2. **Ask Yourself:** Start by asking yourself what your current standards are for how you provide care. Write them down.

   Example of Fall Safety: I expect that my loved one to never fall, and I will ensure constant monitoring and restriction of their movements.

3. **Reflect on the Cost of Perfection:** Consider how striving for perfection impacts your well-being and your relationship with your loved one. Write down these emotional and practical costs.

   Example: Constant monitoring and restriction lead to both of us feeling anxious and restricted. It consumes a lot of mental and physical energy, affecting my overall well-being.

4. **Rewrite your original expectations to a more realistic standard using the Good/Better/Best Framework**

   Good: *I know I can't prevent every fall, but I can reduce the chance of one by implementing safety measures like handrails, non-slip mats, and regular monitoring.*

   Better: *I can ensure my loved one uses mobility aids consistently and maintain clear pathways to reduce fall risks.*

   Best: *I will assist my loved one during all high-risk activities and conduct frequent safety checks and adjustments as needed.*

By reframing perfectionist goals and embracing imperfection, you allow yourself to provide good care (an acceptable but still high standard) for your loved one without overdoing it. As a result, your caregiving becomes more sustainable for yourself and your loved one.

Perspective Shift #3: "I Have to Do Everything Myself" to... "Accepting Help Does Not Make Me a Failure"

Another common limiting belief closely related to perfectionism is the belief that we, as caregivers, need to do everything ourselves. What we don't realize is that the opposite is actually the truth. By accepting help and prioritizing self-care, we can take better care of our loved ones and ourselves. Let's look at Beverley's story as an example.

Beverley's Story: Beverly faced a challenging situation with her husband, who insisted on navigating stairs by himself and walking without a walker at nighttime despite his impaired balance issues. This led to frequent falls and near-misses. She spent many sleepless nights staying awake, listening for any signs of him getting out of bed.

Initially, Beverly struggled with the idea of asking for help. It was her husband, after all, and she believed she should be able to manage independently. However, the lack of sleep had begun to take a toll on her.

One morning, after a particularly restless night, Beverly almost crashed into another car while driving. It was a wake-up call for her, as the strain of continuous vigilance and the fear of his falls had become too much to bear. Realizing she needed to prioritize safety and her well-being, she hired a caregiver to stay overnight.

This decision relieved Beverly. Knowing there was someone to supervise and assist her husband during the night finally allowed her to get the rest she desperately needed. It was a significant step towards accepting the support she required in caring for her husband.

Many caregivers who care for a close loved one may see seeking help as a failure of their ability, and then believe that *they* are a failure.

If this is you, I want to remind you of all the invaluable work you've done so far. Seeking help with dementia care isn't a failure, but a smart, strategic, and intelligent decision. *We are not meant to do all the caregiving, all the time, all by ourselves.* It isn't sustainable, and both you and your loved one will suffer if you continue to hold on to this belief. That's why we need to have a team to help us.

The team can be small (just one other person a few hours a week) or even large (like moving to a facility and having the nursing home staff there to help). The amount and level of help you need will vary (we'll cover more on this in Step 3), but leaning on a team can make all the difference in your caregiving role.

Exercise: Reflecting on Accepting Help

1. **Identify Your Beliefs**: Jot down your current beliefs about seeking help in caregiving. Do you see it as a sign of weakness or strength? Write down any thoughts or emotions that come to mind.
2. **Reflect on Beverly's Experience**: Review Beverly's story and how her perspective shifted when she decided to hire a caregiver. What lessons can you draw from her experience?
3. **List Potential Emotions**: Underneath your beliefs, write down any emotions you associate with accepting help in caregiving. These might include relief, guilt, gratitude, or anxiety.
4. **Potential Benefits**: In another column, list the benefits of accepting help in caregiving. These could include (but are not limited to):
    - Enhanced safety and well-being
    - Reduced stress and burnout for yourself.
    - More time and energy to focus on quality time with your loved one.
5. **Reflect and Reframe**: Consider how reframing any negative beliefs or emotions into more positive and empowering perspectives can support your caregiving journey.

Accepting help is not a sign of weakness but a strategic decision to ensure the best care possible for your loved one and yourself. It can lead to more effective caregiving and a healthier overall caregiving experience.

The Impact of Limiting Beliefs on Your Emotional Health

So far, we've studied three of the most common limiting beliefs that hold us back as care leaders. If you've gone through the exercises, you'll have found ways to reframe these beliefs, and you can even apply these reframing techniques to other beliefs you might be holding on to.

Let me highlight why this work is so important. The longer we hold on to these limiting beliefs, the longer we struggle. And with this struggle, we start to feel emotions like anger, guilt, and sadness. Your emotional well-being is as important as the care you provide.

Anger can stem from the daily frustrations of managing challenging behaviors, the loss of personal time, or the perceived unfairness of the situation. Guilt accompanies caregiving–you may feel guilty for feeling resentful or angry, not doing enough, or taking time for yourself. This guilt is compounded when caregivers feel they must choose between their well-being and the needs of their loved one, leading to a perpetual cycle of self-blame and anxiety.

Feelings of sadness are so, so common. Sadness comes from witnessing the decline of someone we care deeply about, mourning the loss of the person we once knew, and anticipating the grief of future losses. These emotions can create a heavy emotional burden that feels overwhelming at times.

All of these emotions are entirely natural, ones that all of us feel in our caregiving journey, especially with the reality of our loved one's health changes.

However, when these emotions are fueled by limiting beliefs about us and our abilities, they take on a life of their own, quickly leading to overwhelm. Overwhelmed caregivers might feel like they're drowning in responsibilities with no end in sight. In the next chapter, we'll discuss self-care and wellness, which is a requirement of all leaders, particularly when it comes to care leadership.

In this chapter, we explored the transformative journey of caregivers transitioning into care leaders, balancing different perspective shifts. As you grow into your role as a care leader, continue to examine and challenge these limiting beliefs. Only then will you reach your true potential as the leader your loved one needs.

Self-Reflection Questions

1. Describe when you experienced self-doubt in your caregiving abilities. What strategies did you use to build confidence as a care leader?
2. Has it been challenging for you to accept help in the past? Why do you think that is?

Four

Self-Care is a Leadership Requirement

Dear Dr. Thomas,

I've been caring for my mother for the past two years. Unfortunately, she has a tendency to wander around the house without her walker. I can't leave her alone for more than a few minutes because she can be impulsive and has had many falls.

Some days, I don't have the energy to get up and want to lay in bed. But I can't. Between all my responsibilities, I have no time for myself.

At my last doctor's visit, my blood pressure was so high I was started on a new medication. My doctor wants me to lose weight, too. I'm not sure when I'm going to find time to exercise. It just makes me feel so defeated.

I'm not sure what I'm asking for help with. I need help, and I don't know where to start.

Beth

Caregiving Is a Marathon, Not a Sprint

When many women like Beth take on the task of caregiving for a loved one with dementia, it's easy for them to get swept up in the various tasks and responsibilities without stopping to consider the big picture. Remember, caregiving is a marathon, not a sprint. It's a long-term commitment that requires a lot of your energy and time, so it's essential to pace yourself. You'll burn out quickly if you approach this role like a sprint.

This topic is *so important* that I devote an entire chapter in this book to wellness and self-care. These are essential skills all caregivers need. I would say these are requirements for anyone who wishes to be a leader in any area of life. Many business leadership books will discuss the importance of connecting with your team and the client or customer, but true leadership starts with connecting deeply with yourself. Self-care isn't optional; it's a requirement! Without the tools and skills to preserve your energy, protect your health, and safeguard your well-being, your ability to lead effectively will be short-lived.

If you're skimming through this book, you might be tempted to skip this chapter. After all, we've all heard the generic advice on the importance of "wellness" before, right? You might think you'd be better served by reading the chapter on building your care team or learning how to convince your loved one to bathe.

I understand. But hear me out.

As women, we're called to do so much in various spheres of our lives. At home, at work, and in our communities, we juggle countless roles, often under the expectation that we should handle everything cheerfully and without complaint. Society expects us to present ourselves as picture-perfect to the outside world, hiding any of our struggles.

Now, let's add the expectation that women should fill all caregiving roles for their families—whether for elderly parents, ailing spouses, or young children—without seeking help or respite. We're somehow supposed to do it all by ourselves, and asking for a break is often seen as a failure.

Even if we request help, many caregivers struggle to find and access the needed services, not to mention that many of these come at a high cost. Combining societal expectations, heavy responsibilities, and a lack of support creates the perfect recipe for burnout and overwhelm.

I want you to know that it's okay to prioritize your well-being. Prioritizing your wellness through self-care is how you connect deeply with yourself and your needs as a leader. It helps you fill your cup before you pour it out to others. By taking care of yourself, you're ensuring you can continue providing the best care for your loved one. This chapter will give you the tools to sustain your energy and balance. Together, we'll find a path that honors your needs and those you care for.

Understanding Burnout and Its Consequences

In previous chapters, we've discussed the stress of caregiving and its potential impact on you. When these stressors go unaddressed, they can lead to burnout—a state of physical, emotional, and mental exhaustion caused by prolonged and intense stress. For caregivers, burnout can show up in various ways:

- **Physical Symptoms**: Chronic fatigue, frequent illnesses, headaches, and changes in sleep patterns.
- **Emotional Symptoms:** Feelings of helplessness, irritability, and emotional numbness.
- **Cognitive Symptoms**: Difficulty concentrating, memory problems, and decision-making issues.
- **Behavioral Symptoms**: Withdrawal from social activities, neglecting personal responsibilities, and increased use of alcohol or other substances as coping mechanisms.

Some caregivers may not even realize they're burnt out until they develop a serious health issue—like a new diagnosis of depression, anxiety, insomnia, or a chronic medical condition like high blood pressure or diabetes.

Other caregivers might recognize burnout when their close relationships begin to suffer—family and friends distancing themselves due to the chronic emotional stress that accompanies caregiving. This isolation can further exacerbate the caregiver's emotional distress, leaving them feeling even more alone and overwhelmed.

For your loved one with dementia, a burned-out caregiver is less effective and more prone to mistakes. An overtired, under-rested caregiver is more likely to make errors with medication, respond poorly to changes in another person's mood and functioning, and struggle to lead with compassion. It's hard to care with a whole heart when running on empty.

Over time, the chronic stress associated with burnout can lead to a condition known as caregiver syndrome, characterized by severe depression and a sense of hopelessness. This can severely impair your ability to function, sometimes requiring professional intervention and even necessitating you to step down from your role.

There is one more consideration about chronic stress that I want you to pay attention to – a recent study[1] published in 2023 by Wallensten, found that chronic stress and chronic depression can also lead to a higher *risk* of developing dementia, which means that if you don't care for yourself, you are at risk of developing the same illness your loved has!

Have I made my point? Self-Care is Not Optional.

Why Self-Care is a Leadership Requirement

So far, I've talked about the long-term impact of not doing the work of self-care. However, self-care isn't merely a personal necessity but a crucial component of effective leadership in the day-to-day caregiving role.

You may be familiar with the idea of stress hormones. When our bodies are under stress—whether a sudden change or a chronic condition—they release stress hormones like cortisol. These hormones are intended to help us escape from dangerous situations, to fight or flee. However, the front part of our brain, known as the frontal cortex, doesn't like and doesn't respond well to these high stress levels.

The front part of the brain is responsible for key leadership and communication functions, such as choosing the right course of action among multiple choices and responding in a way that considers another person's opinions and perspectives. However, in stressful situations, when cortisol levels are running high, the front part of the brain doesn't operate at its best, and as a result, we don't lead well.

We don't lead ourselves well, we don't lead our care partner well, and we don't lead the team well.

Stressful situations happen daily when caregiving, so knowing how to care for yourself to reduce your stress levels is a critical leadership skill.

Prioritizing your self-care shouldn't make you feel guilty. When you care for your health, you can maintain your energy and build resilience to handle the daily challenges of being a caregiver. Caring for your physical and emotional health enables you to make clear and logical decisions under pressure. Taking time for self-care helps you preserve your sense of self, stay connected to your goals and passions, and bring a more balanced and grounded approach to your caregiving responsibilities.

Before addressing this issue, let's take a moment to understand how significant it is for *you*. Take this short quiz to evaluate how well you care for yourself. Remember to be honest; no one else will be reading these answers!

By identifying areas for growth and seeking out the resources and support you need, you can prevent burnout and find a healthier balance in your caregiving journey. Every step toward better self-care is a step toward being a better care leader.

Exercise: Are You Filling Your Own Bucket?

1. How often do you take time for yourself each day?
   A) Every day
   B) A few times a week
   C) Rarely
   D) Never

2. When was the last time you engaged in an activity you enjoy?
   A) Within the past week
   B) Within the past month
   C) Within the past few months
   D) I can't remember

3. Do you regularly get a full night's sleep (7 – 8 hours)?
   A) Yes, almost every night
   B) Most nights
   C) Sometimes
   D) Rarely or never
4. How often do you exercise or engage in physical activity?
   A) Daily
   B) A few times a week
   C) Once a week
   D) Rarely or never
5. How often do you feel overwhelmed or stressed by your caregiving responsibilities?
   A) Rarely
   B) Occasionally
   C) Frequently
   D) Almost always
6. Do you have a support system (friends, family, support groups) to talk to about your caregiving challenges?
   A) Yes, regularly
   B) Sometimes
   C) Rarely
   D) No support system
7. How often do you neglect your own health needs (doctor appointments, medications) because of caregiving?
   A) Never
   B) Rarely
   C) Sometimes
   D) Often

8. Do you feel guilty when you take time for yourself?
   A) Never
   B) Rarely
   C) Sometimes
   D) Always

Scoring:

- **Mostly A's:** You're doing a great job of filling your own bucket and prioritizing self-care. Keep it up!
- **Mostly B's:** You're aware of the importance of self-care but could benefit from incorporating it more consistently into your routine.
- **Mostly C's:** You may be neglecting your own needs frequently. It's time to reassess and make self-care a priority.
- **Mostly D's:** Your self-care needs significant attention. Remember, taking care of yourself is essential for being an effective caregiver.

If your quiz results indicate that self-care isn't a priority, you might be at risk of burnout. Recognizing the early signs of burnout and taking proactive steps to prevent it are crucial for sustaining your role as an effective caregiver. Next, let's create your self-care plan.

What is a Self-Care Plan?

A self-care plan is your personalized roadmap to maintaining well-being while juggling the demands of caregiving. It's all about your needs, joys, and what helps you recharge. You'll be better equipped to adapt when caregiving circumstances change by crafting a thoughtful and flexible self-care plan.

Here's a closer look at the four critical areas of health that should be part of your self-care plan:

- **Physical Health:** Physical health covers the basics your body needs to function—sleep, hydration, and nutrition. As a caregiver, it's easy to overlook these essentials because of your many responsibilities. You might think it's okay to skimp on sleep or skip meals, but it's not! Your body needs these basics to function at its best. This also includes managing any medical conditions you have, such as taking your medications and attending your doctor's appointments. Your physical health is the foundation of your overall well-being.

- **Social Health:** Humans are social beings who thrive on connections with others. Caregiving can be incredibly isolating. When caregivers get the opportunity to spend time with their family and friends, it's hard to do so without constantly being in "caregiver mode." However, neglecting your social health can lead to a profound sense of isolation that can negatively impact other areas of your life. Make time to nourish your social health—remember that your community is your safety net, providing a helping hand, a shoulder to lean on, or an attentive ear to listen to when you need it most.

- **Emotional Health:** The stresses of caregiving can take a toll on your emotional well-being, leading to feelings of anxiety, anger, and depression. Caring for your emotional health is essential to cultivating positive emotions and safe outlets for negative ones. This might include activities that bring you joy, relaxation techniques, or seeking help from counseling or therapy. Taking care of your emotional health helps you manage the day-to-day challenges of caregiving with greater resilience.

- **Spiritual Health:** When I speak about spiritual health, please note that I'm not asking whether you're religious or not. Spiritual health in this context is about finding meaning and purpose in your life and role as a caregiver, and may or may not be shaped by any religious beliefs you hold. Most importantly, it's about understanding your place in the world and what fulfillment means to you. Cultivating spiritual health involves activities that rejuvenate your spirit and help you find peace and purpose amidst the challenges.

Focusing on these four areas can help you create a comprehensive and flexible self-care plan that supports your well-being and enables you to navigate the demands of caregiving with balance and resilience.

What You Should Include in Your Self-Care Plan

Book Portal Resource Alert!
Get Our Free Self-Care Planner for Caregivers.
Visit your book portal at www.lifecareleadhership.com/dcc

Creating a self-care plan involves identifying what brings you joy, rest, and rejuvenation. Your plan should be unique to you and tailored to nurture your physical, social, emotional, and spiritual well-being. Here are some steps to help you identify what should be in your plan

1. **Reflect on Past Experiences:** Remember moments when you felt genuinely happy and relaxed. What were you doing? Who were you with? Identifying these patterns can help you pinpoint activities that consistently bring you joy.

2. **Identify Your Passions and Interests:** Consider your hobbies and interests. What activities do you look forward to? Whether it's reading, gardening, painting, or walking, incorporating these into your routine can significantly enhance your well-being.

3. **Identify Activities That Support Different Areas of Your Overall Health:** Here are a few suggestions below.

   - **Physical Health:** Exercise such as light walking, getting 7 – 8 hours of sleep each night, and following up with your doctor's recommendations for your health

   - **Social Health**: Contact a friend and schedule a walking date. Join a caregiver support group that meets in person.

- **Emotional Health:** Journal your thoughts and feelings every day to process your emotions. Spend time in nature or engage in an activity that reduces stress.

- **Spiritual Health:** Try getting into the mindfulness habit by watching one of the many free videos available on YouTube.

4. **Find Quick and Easy Activities**: Have a few go-to activities that require minimal effort or planning. If you liked the mindfulness exercises on YouTube, save them to your bookmarks so you can find them quickly when needed. These can be lifesavers when you're short on time but need a quick recharge.

5. **Listen to Your Body and Mind:** Pay attention to how you feel before and after engaging in different activities. Prioritize those that leave you feeling energized and uplifted, and avoid those that drain you.

Implementation Time

Once you've identified the activities that bring you joy and listened to your body's signals, it's time to implement your self-care plan. Your plan should include regular routines and strategies for managing stress when things go off-plan, as they inevitably do.

Your On-Plan Routine: Your On-Plan Routine involves selecting one to two activities from your list and scheduling them throughout the week. Put them on your calendar and treat them as non-negotiable appointments. To set realistic goals, apply the Good/Better/Best framework. For example, "Best" might be exercising for thirty minutes three times a week, while "Good" could be a total of thirty minutes of exercise spread across the week. Aim for the best, but be content with achieving good.

Your Off-Plan Routine: Life can be unpredictable, and there may be times when you fall off your plan. This is where your Off-Plan Routine comes into play. When you find yourself off track, please take a moment to acknowledge it without judgment. Reflect on what caused the disruption and identify any patterns. Then, gently guide yourself back on track by revisiting your goals and making necessary adjustments. Start with small, manageable steps, like one of the quick stress relievers you identified earlier, to rebuild your routine. Remember, being flexible and adapting your plan as needed is okay. The key is to stay committed to your well-being and not be discouraged by setbacks.

Now that we've discussed the importance of self-care in caregiving leadership, it's time to act. Investing in your own well-being enhances your quality of life and strengthens your capacity to be a compassionate and effective caregiver and leader.

Remember, self-care isn't a luxury but a necessity for maintaining balance and resilience in your caregiving role. Take the time to care for yourself and continue caring for others.

Self-Reflection Questions

1. Reflect on a time when you felt overwhelmed by caregiving responsibilities. Did you prioritize your well-being? Why or why not?
2. Consider the societal expectations and cultural norms discussed in the chapter regarding women and caregiving. How have these expectations impacted you?

---

1. Wallensten J, Ljunggren G, Nagar A, Wachtler C, Bogdanovic N, Petrovic P, Carlsson AC. Stress, Depression, and risk of dementia – a cohort study in the total population between 18 and 65 years old in Region Stockholm. Alzheimers Res Ther. 2023 Oct 2;15(1):161. Doi:10.1186/s13195-023-01308-4.

Step 1 Recap

Lead Yourself

As you reflect on your journey through this first part of the book, acknowledge how much you've already grown!

Are You a Care Leader?

In this chapter, we explored the foundational concept of self-leadership. This involves understanding your strengths, weaknesses, and motivations. You can confidently lead by leveraging your strengths and improving your gaps.

Your Caregiving Style

This chapter highlighted the diversity of caregiving approaches and the value of recognizing your own style. Whether you excel in organizing tasks, uplifting spirits, providing nurturing support, or meticulously analyzing care plans, your unique strengths enrich your caregiving journey.

Growth Mindset & Limiting Beliefs

Next, you embraced the transformative power of recognizing your inherent skills and embracing imperfection. You set realistic standards through practical exercises and learned the importance of accepting help when needed.

Self-Care is a Leadership Requirement

Finally, you internalized the crucial role of self-care in sustaining effective caregiving. You learned to invest in self-care practices that preserve your health, prevent burnout, and ensure you can continue to provide compassionate care over the long term.

As you continue reading this book, remember how far you've come! When you're ready, let's turn to Step 2 of our Care Leadership Framework: Leading the Care Partnership.

STEP 2: LEAD THE CARE PARTNERSHIP

Leadership is not about being in charge.
It's about taking care of those in your charge

Simon Sinek

Five

Dementia & the Care Partnership

Dear Dr. Thomas,

For the longest time, I couldn't accept that my sister, Jenny, had early dementia. After all, she only forgot things now and then—wasn't that just normal aging? I forget things sometimes, too.

Everything changed recently when she got lost in our neighborhood last week. The police eventually found her and brought her home, but that episode was a wake-up call for me. I realized I had been in denial, refusing to see Jenny's struggles.

It hit me then that I needed to really be a care leader, like you said, for my sister. But first, I needed to truly understand what was happening with her health. Your training sessions were a game-changer, and I want to thank you for this.

Angie

Understanding the Care Partnership

Welcome to Step 2 of the Confident Care Leadership Framework: Lead the Care Partnership. You've built a solid foundation so far as a care leader, honing your skills to tackle the different challenges that caregiving brings. Now, let's focus on the care partnership and your essential role within it.

Imagine for a moment a big company. Picture it clearly—a vast organization where the head of the company is the CEO, the chief executive officer. The CEO's job is to set the vision and overall plan for the company, which centers on the health, safety, and wellness of their sole client—your loved one with dementia. Next to the CEO's office is the second-in-command, the COO or Chief Operating Officer, whose job is to bring that vision to life by ensuring all day-to-day operations run smoothly.

In this analogy, you are the COO. Your primary responsibility is ensuring the care meets your loved one's needs and enhances their quality of life. Your loved one holds two roles: they are both the sole client and the CEO. However, as their health changes, the CEO will step back and lean on you, the COO, more and more to set the vision and plan.

You need a deep understanding of what your loved one is experiencing to succeed in your task. Let's begin by exploring the nature of dementia and how it impacts their life.

What is Dementia?

Dementia is an umbrella term that describes a range of diseases affecting memory, thinking, and problem-solving. It means that dementia is not just one disease but a group of many different diseases that all have issues with memory and problem-solving to the point where they interfere with everyday life.

Alzheimer's disease is the most common type of dementia, but there are other types, too, each with different features and ways they progress. Let's explore the different types of dementia next.

- **Alzheimer's Disease** is the most common type of dementia. Alzheimer's disease may start with mild memory problems and slowly get worse over time. People with Alzheimer's might forget things, have trouble with language, get confused, and show changes in behavior and mood. As the disease progresses, it can become harder for them to do everyday tasks, and they will need more help from caregivers.

- **Vascular Dementia** occurs when blood flow to the brain is disrupted, often after a stroke or other vascular event. Symptoms can include trouble with judgment, planning, and concentration, but they can vary depending on which part of the brain is impacted. People with vascular dementia may experience stepwise declines in cognitive function, meaning their abilities can worsen suddenly after each vascular event.

- **Lewy Body Dementia** is caused by tiny protein deposits in the brain called Lewy bodies. People with Lewy body dementia might see things that aren't there (visual hallucinations), have problems with movement (like Parkinson's disease), and experience changes in alertness and attention. These symptoms can fluctuate, making it challenging for both the person with dementia and their caregivers. Lewy body dementia can also cause sleep disturbances and difficulty with thinking and reasoning.

- **Frontotemporal Dementia (FTD)** affects the front and side parts of the brain and often starts with changes in personality, behavior, and language rather than memory. People with FTD might act differently, have trouble speaking, or struggle to understand words. Unlike other forms of dementia, FTD can appear earlier in life, between the ages of forty and sixty.

- **Mixed Dementia** happens when someone has more than one type of dementia at the same time, such as both Alzheimer's disease and vascular dementia. Having mixed dementia can make the symptoms more complicated and harder to manage. People with mixed dementia may show a wide range of symptoms from both types, making it essential for caregivers to understand and address the various challenges.

How Is Dementia Diagnosed and Managed?

Doctors can diagnose dementia by examining the patient's medical history, performing physical and neurological exams, and conducting memory tests. Specialists like neurologists, geriatricians, and psychiatrists help with this process. Imaging tests like MRI or CT scans can show changes in the brain that can suggest one of the dementia diagnoses.

Currently, there is no cure for most types of dementia, but there are treatments that can help manage the symptoms and improve the patient's quality of life. Some medications can help slow the progression of the disease and manage symptoms of agitation and anxiety. You must discuss your loved one's symptoms with their doctor to see if one of these medications would be helpful for them. Some new drugs are entering the market that are very promising for the early stages of dementia, bringing hope for a cure in the future. Still, as of the writing of this book, there are no treatments available to cure the late stages of dementia.

Prescriptions and medications are just a *tiny* piece of the plan for caring for someone with dementia. As the primary caregiver, you contribute the *most* by creating a safe environment, providing routine and structure, ensuring their health needs, and providing emotional and social support.

Stages of Dementia: What to Expect Over Time

Understanding how dementia progresses can be complex, but it's important for you as the caregiver to get an idea of how advanced your loved one's condition is and what to expect over time. There are several different staging systems available for dementia, but for simplicity, I will group the stages into four main categories: early, middle, late, and end-stage.

> *A note about stages: Every individual is unique, and it's possible that your loved one doesn't follow the progression from early to middle to late in a stepwise fashion. Use the stages as a rough guideline for what's going on with your loved one and a benchmark for future changes in their health.*

Early-Stage Dementia: In the early stage of dementia, your loved one may experience minor memory lapses, subtle changes in personality, and difficulty with complex tasks. They might need occasional reminders or help to find misplaced objects but can still independently participate in social events with minimal assistance. At this stage, the changes might not be evident to non-family members and could easily be mistaken for just having a bad day.

Middle-Stage Dementia: As dementia progresses to the middle stage, memory loss and confusion increase to the point where others can now see the change. Behavioral changes, such as agitation, anxiousness, or even withdrawal from the usual routine, are also common in this stage. Day-to-day life may involve repeated questions, wandering and getting lost, and difficulty with daily tasks like dressing or cooking. Caregivers might need to establish more structured routines and offer more hands-on assistance.

Late-Stage Dementia: In the late stage, people with dementia start to experience severe cognitive decline. Memory loss is notable, and they might not even recognize close family members. You may notice that it's incredibly challenging to communicate with your loved one because their verbal ability may be limited to a few words or phrases. Daily activities such as eating, toileting, and mobility require full assistance. As a caregiver, at this stage you'll likely need to provide around-the-clock care to maintain their comfort, dignity, and quality of life.

End-Stage Dementia: End-stage dementia represents the final phase of dementia progression. People at this stage depend entirely on others for all parts of care. They may be bedridden and unable to speak with you. They may need to be hand-fed because they can no longer feed themselves. Health complications are expected at this stage, and caregivers may need to make decisions about hospice and comfort care.

As you can see, leading the care partnership requires a deep understanding of your loved one's type and stage of dementia. This knowledge forms the foundation for anticipating their needs and providing practical support throughout their illness. If you're not sure where your loved one would fall amongst the four stages or what type of dementia they have, it's vital that you speak with their physician.

Earlier, I shared the analogy that the care partnership is like the relationship between the CEO, COO, and the client in a company. Another way to think about the care partnership is like a delicate dance, where roles shift over time. Initially, in the early stages of dementia, your loved one may maintain a degree of independence and control; but later in the dance, you become the lead.

In this section, we'll discuss essential parts of your caregiving relationship. First, we'll build awareness of the care partner's needs, discuss how to assess your loved one's changing abilities, and offer practical insights to adapt your caregiving approach accordingly.

Next, we'll focus on the limiting beliefs and relationship mindset shifts that are crucial to succeed in this partnership. Understanding these shifts will help you navigate the evolving roles and responsibilities as dementia progresses.

Communication is the cornerstone of all relationships, and the final chapter in this section addresses common challenges caregivers encounter in this area. From verbal to nonverbal communication strategies, we'll cover how to maintain meaningful connections despite the hurdles presented by dementia.

Remember, as Angie learned through her journey with her sister, each stage of dementia requires flexibility, patience, and a deep understanding of your loved one's needs. As a caregiver transforming into a care leader, you must be ready to grow your knowledge and skill sets. If you go through the exercises and reflection questions in these chapters, I'm confident you'll not only be able to enhance your caregiving skills but also nurture a relationship that respects and supports your loved one's dignity and well-being.

Self-Reflection Questions

1. What type of dementia do you suspect (or know) your loved one has, and how does this understanding influence your caregiving approach? (*It's okay if you don't know, but ask your loved one's doctor for more information.)*

2. Considering the progression of dementia, how do you see yourself changing your approach to adjust to how your loved one's needs will change over time?

Six

Your Care Partner's Needs & Abilities

Dear Dr. Thomas,

I'm feeling so lost and frustrated lately with caring for my dad who has vascular dementia from multiple strokes and uses a wheelchair. I was chatting with my friend Samantha, and she suggested that I try to give my dad simple tasks, like folding laundry. She said it helps her mom, Sarah, stay engaged and gives her a sense of purpose.

So, I decided to try it, but it didn't go as planned. He yelled at me, saying he wasn't a child and didn't need busy work. He even threw the clothes on the floor and refused to talk to me for the rest of the day.

I know that every person with dementia is different, but I don't know where to start. I'm worried about doing more harm than good and further damaging our relationship.

Emily

Understanding Your Loved One's Abilities & Needs

Every care partnership is unique, shaped by the type and stage of dementia and your family's specific circumstances, likes, dislikes, and personalities. This uniqueness can make it challenging for caregivers seeking solutions to everyday problems. Advice that works for one person may not work for you, as Emily discovered when she followed her friend's suggestion, only to have it backfire.

Emily's experience highlights the importance of thoroughly understanding your loved one's abilities and needs before developing a care plan. Each individual with dementia has their own capabilities and challenges, and what works well for one person might not be suitable for another. Conducting a needs and abilities assessment is a crucial first step in increasing your awareness.

A needs and abilities assessment involves evaluating what your loved one requires help with and what they can do independently. This dual focus ensures that the care plan supports their autonomy while addressing their needs.

By the end of this chapter, you'll have conducted a thorough needs and abilities assessment for your loved one. You'll learn how to identify their specific needs and capabilities, allowing you to create a plan that respects their dignity and promotes their independence.

Exercise: Needs & Abilities Quick Assessment

Instructions: For each statement, rate your loved one on a scale from 1-5, 5 being you fully agree with the statement, 1 being that you disagree. (Alternatively, 5 = fully independent, and 1 = fully dependent on someone else to help them with this task). Use this information to identify specific supports and modifications that can improve their quality of life and safety.

1. ______My loved one is able to walk on a level surface without assistance or supervision.
2. ______My loved one moves and transfers independently from bed to chair, or chair to standing, etc.
3. ______My loved one bathes and grooms independently.
4. ______My loved one dresses independently.
5. ______My loved one uses the toilet independently.
6. ______My loved one prepares and eats meals independently.
7. ______My loved one makes decisions and solves problems independently.
8. ______My loved one manages household tasks independently, including cooking and cleaning.
9. ______My loved one manages finances independently.
10. ______My loved one manages medications independently.

The prior assessment is intended to help you get a quick overview of what your loved one can do; but it's essential that, as the care leader, you don't stop at that level but go deeper with a more comprehensive assessment, focusing on four key areas:

1. **Functional Status & Daily Living Activities**: Determine which tasks your loved one can do independently and which ones they need help with. This includes personal hygiene, dressing, eating, and moving around.
2. **Cognitive Abilities:** Look at their memory, problem-solving skills, and ability to follow instructions. This helps you plan activities that are fun and practical for them.

3. **Emotional and Behavioral Needs:** Notice their emotional responses and behavior patterns. Understanding what makes them happy or upset can help create a more comforting environment.

4. **Preferences & Wishes:** Understanding your loved one's preferences and wishes regarding how they wish to be cared for is crucial for all caregivers. This information must guide all the care you provide.

By carefully assessing these four areas, you can develop a plan that respects your loved one's dignity and promotes their well-being. Let's examine all four in greater detail, starting with functional status.

Functional Status: Ability to Perform Daily Living Activities

Evaluating your loved one's functional status means understanding their ability to do basic and complex activities (also known as Activities of Daily Living [ADLs] and Instrumental Activities of Daily Living [IADLs]).

Activities of Daily Living are the basic self-care tasks that a person typically needs to do by themselves. They include:

1. **Bathing**: Can they bathe independently, need supervision, or require full assistance?

2. **Dressing**: Can they dress themselves, need help with buttons, or require full assistance?

3. **Grooming**: Can they brush their hair and teeth, shave, and wash their face independently, or do they need reminders or full support?

4. **Eating**: Can they feed themselves, need help cutting food, or require full feeding support?

5. **Using the Toilet**: Can they use the toilet independently, need supervision, or require full assistance? If they have equipment like a catheter or use disposable underwear – can they manage this by themselves, or do they need help?

6. **Waking & Transferring**: Can they get out of bed or a chair themselves? Can they safely move around their living environment or use an assistive device like a walker or wheelchair? Or do they need someone to be physically present with them at all times to prevent injury?

Instrumental Activities of Daily Living are more complex tasks that a person needs to be able to do to continue independent living. They include:

1. **Managing Finances**: Can they handle money, pay bills, and manage a budget independently, need some supervision, or require full assistance? Have there been issues of missed bills or falling for tele-scammers?

2. **Driving/ Transportation**: Can they drive or use public transport independently, need help planning routes, or require someone to transport them?

3. **Shopping**: Can they make lists, shop for essentials, and handle transactions independently, need help, or require full support?

4. **Meal Preparation**: Can they plan and fully prepare meals independently, need help with specific steps, or require someone to cook for them? If they buy pre-made meals, can they warm them up safely?

5. **Household Tasks**: Can they keep their living environment clean and tidy, and do laundry and dishes? Or will they need someone to help them with these tasks?

6. **Managing Medications**: Can they remember to take them on time, need reminders, or require someone to administer them?

Note that the answers to the above questions on ADLs and IADLs will be very helpful when you get to Step 3: Leading the Care Team, as it will help you determine how much help you'll need and who you need to include in your team.

As part of this assessment, also look at the home environment. Again, being honest and objective is essential; overestimating abilities can lead to safety risks while underestimating can undermine their independence.

Ensuring a safe home environment is critical for the well-being of a person with dementia. This involves checking the home for potential hazards and making necessary changes to prevent accidents. The family home where you grew up may hold a lot of sacred memories, but is it still the *right* environment to meet your loved ones' needs? If not, can it be adapted in any way? Key areas to evaluate include:

- **Fall Risks**: Look for loose rugs and slippery floors, and ensure pathways are clear and well-lit.

- **Kitchen Safety**: Ensure appliances are safe or secured if necessary.

- **Bathroom Accessibility**: Walk through the bathroom with an eye for ease of use—things like toilet seat height, tub showers vs. walk-in showers, and using a shower chair can make a big difference. Also, look to install grab bars (nailed in, never suction type) and non-slip mats.

- **Doors, Steps & Entrances**: Steps and thresholds are common areas where older adults fall—look for places where grab bars can be attached or ramps if needed. If your loved one tends to wander, look for ways to secure doorways.

For Samantha's mother, who could walk around, ensuring pathways were clear and well-lit to avoid falls was crucial. For Emily's father, who used a wheelchair, it was essential to have ramps and wide doorways. Occupational therapists are an excellent resource for ideas–check with your doctor to see if your loved one qualifies for an in-home therapy evaluation.

Cognitive Abilities: Focusing on Strengths

Understanding the cognitive challenges your loved one faces with dementia is crucial for providing adequate care. While it's natural to notice the difficulties they encounter, it's equally important to recognize and nurture their remaining abilities. This approach enhances their quality of life and helps strengthen their existing skills.

Start by observing how they're doing with long-term memory. Typically, individuals with dementia will remember important people and places from their past, although they might struggle with names. Sometimes, individuals may have difficulty recognizing their children because they remember what they looked like as children, not grown-ups. Look for who they consistently recognize.

Do they still recognize close family members and friends? Specific family members? Great! This understanding helps you facilitate social interactions that bring them joy and comfort.

Tip: If your loved one struggles to recognize or remember the names of close family members and friends, please encourage family not to constantly "quiz" your loved one but instead start conversations by immediately reminding them of their name and relationship. For example, don't say, "Mom, do you remember who I am?" Say, "Hi, Mom, it's your daughter, Anna." This approach reduces the stress of having to recall a name out of the blue.

Next, think about short-term memory and learning. How long can they hold onto information to learn new tasks? Can they grasp routines with practice, or do they need ongoing guidance? For example, suppose they can learn to operate a new remote control or remember daily schedules after a few repetitions. In that case, there are a lot of different activities you can try. If their tolerance for learning new routines is low, focus on the activities they enjoy the most. Leveraging these abilities allows you to introduce activities that can slowly stimulate and engage them positively.

Assess their ability to follow instructions and follow a sequence. Can they understand and carry out simple or more complex commands with cues? Adapting tasks to their comprehension level ensures they feel supported and capable, minimizing frustration and maximizing participation.

Memory plays a crucial role in daily life. In the early stages, occasional forgetfulness might mean needing reminders for appointments or assistance with organizing tasks. As dementia progresses, structured routines like labeling drawers, using calendars, and establishing consistent schedules can help reduce confusion and enhance independence.

Focusing on their strengths and abilities can help you create a care plan that respects their dignity and supports their well-being. This positive approach enhances their quality of life and enriches your caregiving experience, making it more meaningful and rewarding for both of you.

Emotional and Behavioral Needs

Understanding and addressing the emotional needs of your loved one with dementia is essential for creating a supportive and nurturing environment. Dementia can bring about significant changes in mood, behavior, and personality, making it crucial to recognize and respond to their emotional state with empathy and sensitivity.

Your loved one may be grappling with cognitive decline and the loss of independence, which can lead to frustration and feelings of inadequacy. As a caregiver, observe their emotional responses to different situations and tasks, noting any patterns of agitation or distress. For example, Emily noticed her father's frustration with tasks he felt were demeaning. She improved his emotional well-being by focusing on activities that respected his dignity and autonomy and reduced distressing episodes.

Exercise: Emotional Needs Assessment & Response

1. **Observation:** Take note of situations or tasks that consistently trigger emotional distress in your loved one.

2. **Adaptation:** Simplify tasks and break them into smaller steps to reduce frustration. Remove triggers from the environment that may cause agitation.

3. **Communication:** Discuss any concerns about emotional health with healthcare providers. They can recommend strategies or therapies to manage depression and anxiety effectively.

Understanding your loved one's natural rhythms throughout the day is crucial. There's a concept known as Diurnal Rhythms, which are natural daily fluctuations in alertness, cognition, and mood that impact all of us. For individuals with dementia, the impact of the time of day may be more notable. For example, mornings may be optimal for mentally stimulating tasks like going to the doctor, while afternoons may require more patience and quieter activities, due to declining cognitive abilities and increased emotional challenges.

> Keep in mind that daily rhythms affect all of us. We all get tired and cranky and regularly need rest and nourishment. When you're stressed-out as a caregiver, this heightens your loved one's stress level, too, so be proactive about implementing the self-care plan we discussed in Step 1 so that you can lead yourself and your loved one.

In the later stages of dementia, individuals may experience increased symptoms of anxiety, agitation, or emotional outbursts. These behaviors often signal underlying discomfort or a need for reassurance, even if they can't verbally express the problem. Caregivers may need to play a detective role, observing behaviors, interpreting cues, and addressing needs promptly to promote calm and security. Agitation can also be worse in new care settings, after medication changes, or after a recent hospitalization, as your loved one needs more time to adapt to a change.

Sundowning is a specific pattern noted in individuals with dementia, where agitated and anxious behaviors become very intense in the early evening hours. Not everyone with dementia develops sundowning symptoms, but when they do occur, they can be intense. Calling out "help me, help me," insisting they want to "go home", increased irritability, or trying to leave are common behaviors you might see. Recognizing when sundowning occurs helps caregivers plan their day and employ calming strategies effectively – ideally, starting calming routines before sundowning takes effect. Sometimes, medications are also needed based on the intensity of the agitation, so be sure to speak with your loved one's doctor if this is required.

Beyond symptoms, formal medical diagnoses of depression and anxiety are also common among individuals with dementia and can exacerbate behavioral symptoms. It's essential to discuss any concerns about your loved one's emotional health with their doctor. Medications or therapeutic interventions may be recommended to help manage these symptoms and improve their overall quality of life.

By tailoring care to their emotional needs and daily rhythms, you can create a supportive environment that enhances their well-being and quality of life. This compassionate approach supports your loved one and enriches your caregiving experience with fulfillment and positivity.

Preferences and Wishes

Understanding your loved one's preferences and wishes is essential for providing compassionate and personalized care. Beyond meeting their basic needs, taking the time to brainstorm what brings them joy and fulfillment allows caregivers to forge deeper connections and nurture their sense of happiness and dignity.

Here's how you can approach this:

Tips: Respecting Their Preferences and Wishes

1. **Identify Their Passions**: Consider the activities or experiences that have historically brought them happiness. Whether it's spending time outdoors, listening to music, or engaging in creative pursuits, these preferences offer meaningful opportunities for interaction and enrichment.

2. **Integrate Activities**: As dementia progresses, engaging in familiar activities becomes increasingly vital. These pursuits offer comfort and familiarity and help preserve their identity and dignity despite cognitive changes.

3. **Respect Their Choices**: Besides activities, they enjoy, explore and respect their preferences regarding care and lifestyle choices. Whether it involves clothing choices, meal preferences, or daily routines, honoring these preferences empowers them.

4. **Discuss Healthcare Directives:** It's crucial to discuss and document advanced healthcare directives, including preferences for medical treatments and end-of-life care. Engage their healthcare provider in these conversations to ensure their wishes are known and respected in future healthcare decisions.

By answering the questions throughout this chapter, you're improving your ability to provide care and becoming a more compassionate leader in your loved one's journey with dementia. Understanding their preferences, needs, and skills helps create a supportive environment promoting happiness, dignity, and quality of life.

This process enhances their daily experiences and strengthens your bond, making caregiving a journey of meaningful interactions and mutual respect.

Self-Reflection Questions

1. How can I apply the insights gained from assessing my loved one's functional, emotional, and cognitive needs to change how I provide care?
2. Have I taken the necessary steps to ensure I'm well-equipped to advocate for my loved one's well-being, including discussing advanced healthcare directives?

Seven

Relationship Mindset & Limiting Beliefs in Care Partnerships

Dear Dr. Thomas,

Lately, I've been grappling with a question that weighs heavily on my heart: Will I lose my husband as I become his caregiver?

His diagnosis of dementia has changed everything. The hardest part is watching his independence slip away. He insists on doing things that aren't safe anymore, like driving, despite the risks. Taking away his car keys was one of my most challenging decisions, and it feels like it's created a divide between us.

We used to talk for hours, finding solace in each other's company. Now, our conversations are often tense and filled with frustration. I worry that as his caregiver, I might lose the best friend and husband I've known for so long.

I really hate this disease,

Jenn

Perspective Shifts in Dementia Care

When a loved one is diagnosed with dementia, it's not just their world that changes—yours does, too. We suddenly find ourselves taking on new roles as care partners, feeling the weight of responsibility while dealing with our emotions, fears, and uncertainties. Navigating the new changes in our relationships with our loved ones is often one of the most challenging parts of transitioning into a care leader.

As we discussed in Step 1, limiting beliefs are deep-seated fears and assumptions that shape our interactions and how we provide care. As we shift from growing ourselves as leaders to understanding and leading the care partnership, new limiting beliefs can emerge and alter our mindset of how we approach caregiving. These beliefs can make it hard to communicate effectively, make decisions together, and maintain the closeness and connection that are so important in our relationships.

I encourage you to embrace a relationship mindset for this stage. A relationship mindset is a view of the care partnership built on the importance of honesty, trust, respect, and communication. By identifying and facing negative limiting beliefs about our relationship head-on, we can start building stronger, more resilient partnerships with our loved ones based on empathy, understanding, and mutual respect.

Three of the most common limiting beliefs that can harm our care partnerships are:

- "My old relationship is gone now that I'm a caregiver."
- "They can no longer make decisions; I have to do it for them."
- "I have to keep them safe at all costs."

Just reading those beliefs feels heavy, doesn't it? Each one has a tiny bit of truth but is buried under loads of untruth. These beliefs can hold back and limit your relationship if left unchecked, adding more emotional stress and negativity. Acknowledging and challenging these limiting beliefs can shift our perspective and approach to caregiving. This will help us foster stronger, more meaningful relationships with our loved ones.

Let's discuss these beliefs in more detail and see how we can overcome them together.

Perspective Shift#1: "My Old Relationship Is Gone Now That I'm a Caregiver" to... "My Relationship Has Changed, But the Love Still Remains"

The fear of becoming a caregiver and how it might negatively change a relationship is a serious concern. Whether you're a spouse or a child, stepping into the role of a caregiver can be emotionally challenging. Jenn's journey with her husband shows how hard it can be to move from being a partner to a caregiver. As dementia progresses, their relationship changes a lot, making it hard to keep the same level of closeness and connection.

For spouses like Jenn, this fear often centers around losing the equal, romantic relationship they've built over the years. Watching a partner's independence fade and taking on more responsibilities is tough. The daily realities of caregiving can feel like they're overshadowing the intimacy and shared history that made the relationship special.

On the other hand, when children become caregivers for their parents, they face different challenges. There's often a fear of role reversal. The child now must take on responsibilities that the parent once held. This shift can bring feelings of guilt, sadness, and inadequacy. Parents may struggle with losing their independence and the reversal of roles, while children bear the emotional weight of becoming the primary decision-makers and protectors. It's hard for parents to see themselves as a burden and for children to see their strong, guiding parents in a vulnerable state.

However, amidst all these changes and challenges, remember that the core of these relationships—love and companionship—has to remain strong. Yes, things are changing, and yes, these changes are hard, but the foundation of your bond needs to stay solid. Even in the later stages of dementia, when recognition may falter, the warmth of your shared history will continue to strengthen you.

To help reframe this limiting belief, let's look at ways to keep and deepen your connection with your loved one throughout their dementia journey. Despite the challenges, many opportunities exist to create joy, laughter, and connection.

Exercise: Recognizing Your Relationship

1. **Identify Special Moments**: Write down three moments in the past week where you felt connected to your loved one. This could be a smile they gave you, a shared laugh, or a quiet moment holding hands.
2. **Recall Memories:** Share a favorite memory with your loved one. Even if they can't recall it, the act of sharing can bring you closer and remind you of the bond you share.
3. **Celebrate Small Wins:** Acknowledge and celebrate the small victories. Did your loved one recognize you today? Did they respond positively to something you said or did? These moments are precious and worth celebrating.

Focusing on these simple relationship reminders can help preserve and strengthen the unique bond you share with your loved one. Yes, things are different, but your relationship still exists at its core and can grow in new ways.

Perspective Shift# 2: "They Can No Longer Make Decisions; I Have to Do it for Them." to... They Can Still Express a Choice, and I Can Remember Their Past Decisions for Them"

When a loved one has dementia, making decisions can be really tough. It's like walking through a fog, trying to understand their needs and preferences as they change. Let's look at Maya's story to see how she navigated this challenging limiting belief around decision-making with her mom.

Maya's Story: Maya faced a big decision: whether to accept hospice care for her mom. Her mom had end-stage dementia and couldn't communicate with her anymore.

Maya felt overwhelmed, worried she wasn't doing the right thing, and didn't have the help she needed to care for her properly. Multiple family members were calling and pressuring her to make conflicting choices that didn't feel right to her, adding to her stress.

Then, Maya began to reframe her thinking. She remembered how her mom was never fond of going to the hospital and how she always seemed most comfortable when cared for at home. By leaning on these memories, Maya realized she could still let her mom guide her in this decision. Even though her mom couldn't make complex decisions anymore, Maya could trust her understanding of her mom's past preferences to lead her.

Maya decided to consider hospice care, knowing it could provide comfort and allow her mom to stay in the familiar and loving environment of home. The visiting nurses and the support she would receive from the hospice team was exactly the kind of care her mom would prefer, rather than making the trip to the emergency room again.

This perspective helped Maya feel more confident and connected, knowing she was honoring her mom in the best way possible.

It's important to remember that in the early stages of dementia, people will still be able to make a lot of decisions, like where they want to live or how they wish to prepare their advanced directives. But as dementia advances, this ability slowly fades, and decision-making becomes more limited, especially when it comes to complex medical and financial decisions. Over time, as the caregiver for a loved one with dementia, there will be many decisions you'll have to make on their behalf. As the leader of a care partnership, however, your choices should always reflect your knowledge of what your loved one would want.

The following exercise will help you get a clearer understanding of these wishes.

Exercise: Reflecting on Prior Wishes and Stated Preferences – When your Loved One Can No Longer Tell You.

1. **Remembering Prior Wishes:** Think about a time when your loved one expressed their preferences or wishes before dementia affected their ability to communicate clearly.
2. **Reviewing Advanced Directives:** If your loved one has advanced directives or written instructions about their care preferences, review them carefully. Consider how these directives align with their current needs and circumstances.
3. **Discussing with Others:** Talk to other family members or close friends who knew your loved one well before dementia. They might offer insights or memories that could help you make decisions that honor your loved one's wishes.

By taking these steps, you can better navigate decision-making with empathy and confidence, honoring your loved one's autonomy and ensuring their care reflects their values and preferences. Remember that even if they can't make complex decisions now, they can still express a choice, and you, as their caregiver, can use the memory of their past decisions to guide you.

Perspective Shift #3: "I Have to Keep Them Safe at All Costs" to... "I Can Balance Safety while Prioritizing Autonomy and Dignity for My Loved One"

In caregiving for loved ones with dementia, another common limiting belief centers around the overwhelming need to prioritize safety at all costs. But what happens when this pursuit compromises the dignity and self-worth of those we care for?

> *Betty's case:* Betty faced a daunting challenge when her father, diagnosed with frontotemporal dementia, began exhibiting impulsive behavior. Despite her best efforts to keep him safe, he would frequently attempt to get out of his chair or bed without assistance, often resulting in falls and injuries. Additionally, he struggled with incontinence, which further complicated matters.
>
> The instinct to prioritize her father's safety was deeply ingrained for Betty. She believed that she had to do whatever it took to prevent him from harming himself, even if it meant compromising his dignity in the process. Fearing for her father's safety, Betty turned to the internet for solutions. She researched physical restraints to keep him secured in chairs, hoping to prevent accidents.
>
> However, deep down, she felt conflicted and troubled by the idea. Betty knew that physical restraints could compromise her father's dignity and worsen his agitation. In addition, as she witnessed the toll that constant supervision and intervention took on her father's sense of autonomy and self-worth, Betty began to question the balance between safety and dignity in caregiving.

This common dilemma among caregivers highlights the tension between ensuring physical safety and respecting the autonomy and dignity of loved ones with dementia. While safeguarding their well-being is crucial, it's equally important to honor their desire for independence and preserve their sense of dignity.

Exercise: Reframing the Belief of Safety vs. Independence:

1. **Is there an Unmet Need Driving the Unsafe Behavior?** Ask if there are specific triggers for behaviors like attempting to move independently or experiencing discomfort? In Betty's case, she realized that many of her father's attempts to get out of the chair were related to his urge to urinate – he was actually trying to meet a biological need, and an emotional desire to prevent having an accident.

2. **Promote Autonomy Where Possible:** Look for opportunities to promote autonomy and empower your loved one's independence. Are there tasks they can still manage with some support or guidance?

3. **Holistic Care Approach:** Take a holistic approach to caregiving that considers both physical safety and emotional well-being. How can you create a safe environment that respects their independence and choices? This may involve modifying the home environment, establishing routines, or exploring assistive devices that promote independence while ensuring safety. Betty opted to include the help of in-home physical and occupational therapists who helped her strategize and meet her father's care needs.

By reframing your approach to caregiving, you can foster a supportive and empowering environment that enhances your loved one's quality of life while addressing their safety needs. Embracing their autonomy and dignity ensures that they continue to feel valued and respected throughout their dementia journey.

Impact of Trust on Leadership

In this chapter, we've explored three fundamental perspective shifts foundational to your care partnership: how you view the relationship, make decisions, and balance safety and independence. For all three, trust is the crucial element that forms the cornerstone of your partnership. When you and your loved one with dementia don't have that inner foundation of trust, it's hard to give and receive care. This is why holding on to these limiting beliefs can be so dangerous—they erode the trust in the relationship, leading to misunderstandings and conflict.

For example, if a caregiver believes that their loved one with dementia is incapable of making any decisions and insists on controlling every aspect of their life, it can breed frustration and resentment. This lack of trust can erode the caregiver's authority over time, making it hard to provide compassionate care. Similarly, if a caregiver prioritizes safety above all else and imposes strict restrictions on their loved one's freedom and independence, it can foster feelings of helplessness and disempowerment.

Through the stories of Jenn, Maya, and Betty, we've seen how caregivers can overcome these limiting beliefs, especially by remembering that trust and compassion are the most vital tools in your toolbox. In the next chapter, we'll focus on understanding communication changes with dementia to help you improve and strengthen your connection with them.

Self-Reflection Questions

1. How has your relationship with your loved one changed since becoming their caregiver? Can you identify moments when you strongly connected with them despite these changes?

2. What actions can you take to build or rebuild trust in your caregiving relationship? How can you ensure that trust remains a cornerstone of your care partnership?

Eight

Communication Changes in Dementia

Dear Dr. Thomas,

I know you focus on women, but I hoped you could advise my wife, Lillian, and me.

When we are with friends, my wife always appears. She interacts and laughs with others and seems at ease. No one else has seemed to notice a significant change.

However, when it's just the two of us, I can tell she is different. She often refuses suggestions like taking a bath or taking medications. She struggles to follow a deeper conversation or a complicated task. She may repeat questions and seems fixated on specific topics that are easier for her.

Why is there such a difference, and how do I help her?

A concerned husband,

Louis

How Communication Changes with Dementia

Communication is at the heart of every relationship and is the connecting factor that links people together, helping them understand and support each other. Effective communication is key to caregiving, especially for those with dementia. It shapes how caregivers and their loved ones interact and feel.

In this chapter, we'll explore how communication abilities change with dementia and how to handle common challenging scenarios. While someone in the early stages of dementia might chat easily in social settings, their ability to understand complex ideas and remember things can be notably different in private settings. Louis saw this with his spouse, who struggled with complex conversations and understanding information, showing deeper interaction challenges.

For a moment, let's take a step away from dementia care and talk about communication. We all communicate daily, and it may feel effortless – but it's a very complex skill! If you think about it, communication involves taking in what the other person said, including visual and auditory information, processing it, formulating a response, and then expressing it. This goes back and forth between two or more people in conversations and requires us to integrate what we hear and see with our thoughts, opinions, and memories. For communication to be clear, all of these things have to happen quickly and without interruptions.

In dementia, these interactions become more complicated because cognitive issues can disrupt the flow of information in and out. Even though hearing might be okay, difficulties understanding language, processing information, and expressing thoughts can be challenging. Let's investigate some of these changes in greater depth.

Hearing and Language Processing Challenges

Let's start by thinking about how we communicate, especially regarding auditory/verbal information, i.e. – talking and listening. When we talk to someone, we rely heavily on what we can hear and understand. There are two key steps here: (1) hearing the words and sounds and (2) processing what the sounds mean.

Hearing ability is simply whether a person can hear sounds around them. Hearing loss is not a typical feature of dementia, but it's common for many older adults. In fact, sometimes severe hearing loss can mimic dementia—but the problem is with the ears, not the brain! If your loved one struggles with conversations, you must check for hearing loss with an audiologist and use hearing aids if needed. Hearing aids can make sounds louder and clearer, helping the person hear better.

But hearing is just the first part. The second and sometimes more challenging part is understanding what those sounds mean. People with dementia might hear you perfectly but still struggle to know what you're saying. This is because their brain has trouble processing spoken language.

For someone with dementia, it's like they only hear every third or fourth word you say. Imagine trying to make sense of a sentence where you only catch bits and pieces. For example, if you say, "Would you like to go get a sandwich and eat in the park?" they might only catch "Would ..to...and...park?" They must guess the rest, which can be really tough. This makes longer and more complex conversations especially difficult.

Communication Tips When Your Loved One Has Hearing Concerns

- **Speak Slowly and Clearly:** This gives the person more time to process your words.
- **Use Simple Language:** Shorter, more straightforward sentences are easier to understand.
- **Pause Often:** Give them time to catch up and think about what you said.
- **Add Visual Cues:** Show them what you're talking about or demonstrate actions.

Visual Impairment and Focus

A lot of our communication occurs visually. We look at the person we are talking to, see that they're speaking, and read their facial expressions and gestures. As we get older, our vision may decline, but for those with dementia, this can be even more noticeable. This makes it harder for them to talk and eat simultaneously or prepare for the day.

As individuals with dementia age, their visual field—the total area they can see clearly at one time—becomes narrower. This narrowing of the visual field means they might not see objects or people unless they're directly in front of them. It's like they're looking through blurry binoculars all the time. As a result, they may miss things around them. For instance, if you place a plate of food to their side or try to talk to them from an angle, they might not notice you (especially if they also have hearing loss) or the food at all (leading to untouched food trays). Understanding these changes helps caregivers approach and communicate more effectively. Here are a few tips you can try:

Communication Tips When Your Loved One Has Vision Concerns

- **Positioning During Conversations**: Sit or stand in front of their main field of vision during conversations. This direct line of sight helps them focus on your face and mouth movements, making it easier to understand what you're saying.
- **Placing Objects**: Always place objects, like food or drinks, directly in their line of sight. If you put a plate of food to the side, they might not see it and could miss mealtime entirely. Centering items in front of them ensures they notice and can interact with these objects.
- **Using Large Print and High Contrast**: Use large print and high-contrast colors for any written communication, such as notes or labels. This makes reading easier and reduces the strain on their vision. Simple, bold fonts on plain backgrounds are best.

Thought Processing Challenges

Once your loved one with dementia can see and hear you, they still need to process the information and decide on a response. Individuals with dementia often face challenges in thought processing, which can significantly impact how they communicate. As dementia progresses, cognitive functions such as problem-solving, cause-and-effect reasoning, and abstract thinking may become more impaired.

Decision-Making and Complex Tasks: Individuals with dementia may struggle to make decisions or solve problems that require planning and organization. Tasks that once seemed simple, like managing finances or following a recipe, can become overwhelming and confusing because of all the steps that must be followed correctly in the correct sequence. This difficulty can impact their ability to express their needs or preferences clearly.

Short-Term Memory and Cause and Effect: Remembering new things, events, or actions is particularly difficult with dementia. In addition, people with dementia may have trouble understanding cause-and-effect relationships or anticipating the consequences of their actions.

This can lead to what we may assess as impulsive or risky behaviors. For instance, they might forget to turn off the stove after cooking and wander away—this might be because they forgot they were cooking in the first place or have forgotten that a hot stove can lead to fires. Communicating safety instructions or reminders becomes a challenge in such situations.

Abstract Thinking and Comprehension: The loss of abstract thinking abilities affects their comprehension of complex concepts and conversations. They might struggle to follow the plot of a movie or understand metaphors and figurative language. Conversations must become more straightforward and to the point. As a result, the natural poetic flow of a conversation can be lost, leading to frustration and social isolation for both the individual with dementia and their caregivers.

Here are a few tips to help your loved one if they are struggling with processing issues:

Communication Tips When Your Loved One Struggles With Processing Thoughts

1. **Simplify Decisions:** Help them make decisions by offering limited choices. Instead of asking open-ended questions like, "What do you want to eat?" you could ask, "Would you like chicken or fish for dinner?" This approach reduces the cognitive load and makes it easier for them to choose.
2. **Break Down Tasks:** Simplify complex tasks into smaller, manageable steps. Instead of giving them a list of instructions all at once, break it down. For example, if they're getting dressed, guide them step-by-step, like "First, put on your shirt," then "Now, put on your pants."
3. **Use Clear and Direct Language:** Avoid using abstract language or metaphors. Instead, use clear, straightforward language that they can easily understand. For example, instead of saying, "It's raining cats and dogs," you could say, "It's raining very heavily."
4. **Patience and Repetition**: Be patient and prepared to repeat information as needed. Allow them extra time to process what you've said and respond. Reassure them that it's okay to take their time.

Expressive Difficulty & Word Finding Challenges

Now that your loved one has processed their thoughts, they need to communicate their response to you. However, individuals with dementia often face word-finding difficulties, which can cause breakdowns in communication.

Recalling Words and Phrases: Individuals with dementia often pause mid-sentence as they try to remember a word. This can be frustrating for them and confusing for others, as it seems like they suddenly stopped the conversation. Sometimes, they might use a word that sounds similar but doesn't fit the context. In other cases, they may struggle to remember a loved one's name, which can be deeply upsetting for close family members.

Nonsensical Speech: When they can't find the right word, they might use words or phrases that don't make sense. In advanced stages of dementia, you may hear more sounds than actual words. This can make it hard to understand what they're trying to communicate.

Filling in the Blanks: Sometimes, the person with dementia will fill in the blanks of their missing memory with an invented false memory. They may tell you all about what they did that day like going to the bank, talking to a friend, etc., when they did none of those things. It's not that they're deliberately lying, but that they genuinely believe this happened. This phenomenon, known as confabulation, is common in dementia related to heavy alcohol use, but is also seen in other types of dementia.

Here are a few strategies you can try:

Communication Tips When Words are Hard to Find

1. **Patience and Support**: Give them plenty of time to express themselves without feeling rushed or pressured. Let them know it's okay to take their time. Interrupting their train of thought will only add to their frustration and confusion as they try to express themselves.

2. **Use Visual Aids**: Communication boards, picture cards, or even visual aids can be very helpful. These tools provide prompts that assist in conveying messages and ideas, especially for those who struggle with verbal expression. For example, holding a glass of water when asking if they're thirsty helps them process what you're saying to them, linking the question with the task at hand.

3. **Repeat and Rephrase:** If they can't find the right word, repeat their sentence back to them or gently rephrase it. For instance, if they say, "I want the thing," and they're in front of their television, you might ask, "Do you want the TV remote?"

Musical Memory & Social Graces: A Pleasant Surprise in Dementia Care

One fascinating part of dementia is that although language ability decreases over time, musical memory is usually retained for a long time. People with dementia often remember childhood songs, melodies, prayers, and rhythms, showing how deeply music is stored in our brains. Caregivers often see their loved ones tapping their feet, humming along, or singing old songs, which can bring comfort and joy.

Caregivers can use music to communicate without words. Playing familiar songs during meals or activities can create a calming atmosphere and help express emotions without needing to talk.

Alongside musical memory, simple social conversations and greetings usually remain easy for them, like saying, "Hello, how are you?" Despite struggles with deeper conversations, individuals may still enjoy light discussions and social interactions. This familiarity helps them feel connected and normal but can also be why early dementia symptoms can be hidden from people we don't interact with regularly.

However, do recognize that while music and social niceties may be retained, understanding complex instructions and having detailed conversations can be challenging for people with dementia. This discrepancy can make it harder for family members to accept that their loved one has a diagnosis of dementia.

Non-Verbal Communication

Nonverbal communication plays a vital role in dementia care, especially when verbal abilities start to decline. Even as spoken language becomes challenging, individuals with dementia can still express their needs through tone of voice, facial expressions, and body language as long as you watch carefully. Caregivers who understand these nonverbal cues can better support their loved ones' needs.

For example, you may be able to tell just by observing your loved one's body language when they're getting angry or frustrated, or perhaps need a change insetting. A sudden change in behavior—like becoming more agitated, throwing things, etc.—should prompt a check to see whether something's changed in their health and well-being. Perhaps they're in pain, and this is how they're communicating the issue with you.

Here are some practical tips for interpreting and responding to nonverbal cues in dementia care:

Communication Tips When Your Loved One Can No Longer Speak

1. **Observe Facial Expressions:** Pay attention to changes in facial expressions, such as smiles, frowns, or furrowed brows. These subtle shifts can convey happiness, frustration, confusion, or discomfort.

2. **Listen to Tone of Voice:** Notice tone, pitch, and volume variations. A gentle tone can soothe, while a sharp tone might cause agitation. Speak calmly and reassuringly to promote a sense of security.

3. **Respond to Body Language:** Watch for gestures, posture changes, and restless movements. Pacing might indicate restlessness or a need for activity, while fidgeting might suggest discomfort.

Please don't forget that non-verbal communication goes both ways! Even when words are hard to grasp, your loved one with dementia can still sense emotions conveyed through *your* tone of voice and facial expressions. They may not understand the details of what you are saying, but they can perceive whether you are happy or mad at them based on how you interact with them. This highlights the importance of maintaining a calm and caring approach during interactions, as these emotional signals greatly influence their sense of security and well-being.

Applying Communication Lessons to Challenging Situations

As dementia progresses, communication breakdowns become common and can impact how we keep our loved ones safe, healthy, and happy. Understanding these changes discussed above is crucial because it provides insight into how interactions evolve. Let's discuss three specific types of challenging situations:

Case Study: Managing Dangerous Behaviors & Stopping Driving

> Case: Jen's father, who was diagnosed with dementia, insisted he could still drive, even after his physician revoked his license for safety reasons. Despite repeated discussions, Jen faced constant resistance and frustration as her father struggled to understand why he could no longer drive. Jen finally moved his car to her house to prevent him from driving, but then found out later that he had a friend drive him to the dealership, where he bought himself a new car.

This situation highlights a common challenge in dementia care where individuals may lack awareness of their limitations and the associated safety risks.

Several factors contribute to this communication breakdown:

- **Lack of Awareness:** Individuals with dementia often lose insight into their abilities and limitations, making it challenging for them to recognize that their driving skills have declined.

- **Impaired Safety Awareness and Cause & Effect Reasoning:** Dementia can affect judgment and the ability to assess risks, leading to behaviors like insisting on driving despite being unsafe.

- **Memory Issues:** Individuals may forget previous discussions about not driving, resulting in repeated confrontations and misunderstandings.

Talking about stopping dangerous behaviors, like driving, with someone who has dementia can get heated quickly. It's important to understand that this is a complicated issue. Even if a doctor says they can no longer drive and revokes their license, keeping them away from the car is another problem. Recognizing this helps you approach the situation with kindness and understanding.

Be ready for these conversations to happen more than once. It's normal to discuss stopping dangerous behaviors many times. Try to be patient and consistent each time, gently reminding them why it's necessary. Always stay calm and compassionate.

When you talk about stopping these behaviors, use clear and simple words. Explain the safety concerns and risks plainly, without complicated details that might confuse them. Remember, they might not fully understand the dangers they're facing, but they may fully appreciate that you are taking away their independence.

Instead of focusing on what they can't do, offer safe alternatives. For example, if driving is the issue, find other ways for them to get around, like arranging rides or using transportation services. This helps shift the focus from losing independence to finding safe and reliable ways to stay mobile.

Also, make their environment as safe as possible. This might mean hiding car keys, changing things around the house, or using safety devices. A supportive and secure home can help prevent them from doing risky things.

Case Study: Encouraging Needed Behaviors Such as Showering.

Encouraging individuals with dementia to engage in essential self-care tasks, such as showering or taking medication, can be challenging and even met with resistance or outright refusal. This situation often leads to frustration and tension for both caregivers and their loved ones and is a common struggle in the middle stages of dementia. Let's review Mary's situation:

> Case: Mary is a devoted daughter who cares for her mother, who has dementia. One of Mary's biggest challenges is getting her mother to shower regularly. Every time Mary tries to encourage her mother to bathe, she's met with excuses, resistance, and sometimes outright refusal. Mary's mother often insists that she has already showered or doesn't need to, even when it's clear she hasn't. This constant struggle leaves Mary feeling frustrated and helpless, unsure how to ensure her mother's hygiene while maintaining a positive and loving relationship.

The breakdown in communication in these scenarios can stem from several factors:

- **Lack of Awareness:** Individuals with dementia may not understand the importance of the task or may forget why it's necessary, leading to resistance or refusal.

- **Inability to Express Discomfort:** They might have valid concerns, such as feeling cold, fearing a fall, or being overwhelmed, but struggle to communicate these issues effectively.
- **Feeling Infantilized:** Being reminded to perform basic tasks can undermine their sense of independence and dignity, causing them to resist out of frustration or a desire to maintain autonomy.

Establishing trust is crucial when encouraging a loved one with dementia to engage in self-care tasks. Approach the person with kindness and understanding, validating their feelings and concerns. Explain the task calmly and respectfully, ensuring they feel listened to and respected. Use gentle language and a soothing tone to help them feel at ease. Show empathy by acknowledging their emotions, saying, "I understand this might be uncomfortable, but I'm here to help you."

Take time to understand why they might be resistant. For instance, they may be afraid of falling, are feeling cold, or don't understand the steps needed in the bathroom anymore. Address these concerns directly by ensuring the bathroom is warm enough, providing non-slip mats and handrails for added safety, or breaking down the task into smaller, more manageable steps. You could also use adaptive equipment, like a shower chair, to make the process more comfortable and safer for them.

Creating a consistent daily routine for self-care tasks is also helpful. Incorporate familiar cues and gentle reminders to make the process smoother. This could mean establishing a specific time each day for the task to become a predictable part of their routine. Use visual aids like a calendar or pictures to reinforce the schedule. Additionally, make the experience more enjoyable by integrating activities they like, such as playing their favorite music during shower time or using scented soaps they prefer. These small touches can transform a potentially stressful activity into a more pleasant and calming experience.

And finally, it's essential to pick your battles when caring for someone with dementia. Not every issue needs to be addressed immediately or with the same level of urgency. Prioritize tasks based on their impact on health and safety. For example, if your loved one resists showering daily but is willing to bathe every other day or at least twice a week, compromising might be okay. This approach reduces stress for you and your loved one, making caregiving more manageable. If they're adamant about wearing the same outfit two days in a row, but it's clean, it's probably best to let it go. Save your energy for more critical issues, like taking medications on time or attending medical appointments.

Case Study: Identifying Issues When Verbal Communication Is Limited or Absent

As dementia progresses to the late stages, verbal communication often diminishes, leaving caregivers to figure out their loved one's needs and emotions through alternative means. Let's review Annmarie's situation with her grandmother.

> Case: As Annmarie's grandmother's dementia progressed, she became nonverbal and started moaning and muttering incomprehensible sounds. Annmarie found it increasingly difficult to understand what her grandmother's vocalizations meant, whether they signaled pain, discomfort, or confusion. This inability to communicate effectively left Annmarie frustrated and unsure how best to assist her grandmother, highlighting the significant challenges of caregiving in such situations.

In such situations, communication breakdowns can stem from several key challenges:

- **Loss of Verbal Abilities:** As dementia advances, individuals may lose their capacity to speak clearly or coherently. They may struggle to find words or phrases, leading to incomplete or unclear communication.
- **Difficulty Interpreting Nonverbal Cues:** Caregivers may encounter difficulties in interpreting nonverbal signals such as facial expressions, body language, or changes in behavior. These cues can be subtle and require careful observation to understand.
- **Unmet Needs:** When verbal communication is compromised, essential needs like hunger, pain, or discomfort may go unrecognized. This can lead to increased agitation or distress as the person struggles to convey their needs effectively.

When caring for individuals with dementia, paying close attention to nonverbal cues such as body language, facial expressions, and behavioral changes is essential. These cues can offer valuable insights into their emotional state and physical comfort. For instance, signs of discomfort may manifest as restlessness, agitation, or facial grimacing. Observing these subtle cues allows caregivers to identify potential sources of discomfort, whether physical discomfort like pain or discomfort stemming from environmental factors such as noise or lighting.

Caregivers should be vigilant in noting changes in behavior that could indicate discomfort or distress. For example, sudden agitation or withdrawal from activities they typically enjoy may signal discomfort that needs addressing. It's essential to approach these observations with empathy and patience, acknowledging that people with dementia may not always be able to verbalize their feelings.

Beyond body language, understanding facial expressions can provide significant clues. A furrowed brow, clenched jaw, or wide eyes may indicate pain or discomfort. Caregivers should also consider environmental factors contributing to discomfort, such as room temperature, uncomfortable seating, itchy clothes, or unfamiliar surroundings.

As we wrap up this chapter on communication and leading the care partnership in dementia caregiving, let's review what we've covered. In this chapter, you've not only gained insights into what changes are occurring within your loved one that impact their ability to communicate but also learned how to respond to those needs with specific strategies. We also covered three common issues: stopping dangerous behavior, encouraging a needed behavior they're resisting, and nonverbal communication issues.

Self-Reflection Questions

1. How have I observed communication changes in my loved one since their dementia diagnosis?

2. Reflecting on my current approach, what adjustments should I make to become a better care leader?

Step 2 Recap
Lead the Care Partnership

It's time to reflect on your journey as a care leader and see how you've grown over the last few steps!

Dementia & the Care Partnership

In this introductory chapter, you deepened your understanding of dementia—its types such as Alzheimer's, vascular dementia, Lewy body dementia, and frontotemporal dementia—and its progression through the four stages. With this knowledge, you're better prepared to anticipate and meet your loved one's evolving needs.

Your Care Partner's Needs & Abilities

This chapter emphasized the importance of personalized assessments for your loved one with dementia. It guided you in assessing functional status, cognitive abilities, emotional needs, and preferences. As a result, you gained greater awareness of how to best help your loved one in your care partnership.

Relationship Mindset & Limiting Beliefs in Care Partnerships

This chapter revealed the profound shifts you need to make in caregiving relationships and challenged you to confront any fears of losing the connection you once had with your loved ones by embracing a relationship mindset.

Communication Changes in Dementia

Next, we discussed how dementia alters communication abilities and impacts our interactions with loved ones, especially during challenging times. We explored effective communication strategies and how to tackle issues like stopping driving, encouraging needed behaviors like bathing, and what to do when your loved one is no longer verbal.

But we're not done yet; so please turn the page to start Step 3!

STEP 3: LEAD THE CARE TEAM

Alone, we can do so little;
together, we can do so much.

Helen Keller

Nine

Why You Need a Team

Dear Dr. Thomas,

I've spent years caring for my husband as he's battled Parkinson's disease and now lung cancer.

Recently, his condition has become more challenging, and I've finally realized I need help. I've been doing it all alone for so long that I'm unsure where to begin.

How do I figure out how much help we need and who would best fit us?

I feel lost in this new phase of needing assistance after being the sole caregiver for so long.

Thank you so much for all your help,

Theresa

Becoming a Team Leader

Welcome to Step 3: Lead the Care Team. As you've read this book, each section has built on the last, improving your leadership skills – from caring for your loved one as an individual to working together in a partnership and now leading a team of caregivers.

Throughout this journey, you've likely had moments when you learned important things about yourself and your relationship with your loved one who has dementia. These moments aren't just facts but deep realizations that have shaped how you care.

I know how much care and effort you've put into looking after your loved one. Your journey shows how strong and determined you are. But as your loved one's needs change, there comes a time when one person can't do everything alone anymore, just like my client Theresa learned.

In this third step of the Confident Care Leader Framework, it's time to put those realizations into practice. Leading a care team means stepping out of your comfort zone. It means taking on new responsibilities and facing challenges with bravery and kindness.

Moving from being the primary caregiver to leading a team is a significant change. It means moving from doing things by yourself to working together with others to make sure your loved one gets all the care they need.

As you take on this new role, you'll face challenges that will test your skills, patience, and strength. You'll need to learn new ways to talk to people, ask for help, and ensure that your loved one gets the best care possible, both physically and emotionally.

Why You Need a Team

Many caregivers struggle to consider a team; after all, they've been managing pretty well so far, right? If this is you, I want you to reconsider.

Dementia care will get more complicated in the late and advanced stages, requiring more hands-on caregiving like dressing and bathing. If your loved one is still mobile, they may need constant supervision to prevent injury. All of this together means that caregiving may become a full–time 24/7 job—too much for one individual to manage while also trying to take care of their own needs and health.

We aren't meant to do this alone; we need a village around us, people with different strengths that we can rely on. I recommend that you build this village slowly but early on, as it takes time for you and your loved one to adapt and adjust.

In my experience, once you have the right team around, you'll see that they're a huge asset not only to your caregiving abilities but also your own well-being. Now you have the time and energy to spend time with your loved one as their loved one, which is so important to maintaining that relationship.

Understanding Your Roles and Responsibilities

What does being a care team leader really mean? It's more than just a title—it's a transformative role where you shift from being the sole caregiver to orchestrating a team effort involving doctors, nurses, therapists, private aides or support workers, and family members, all rallying together for your loved one's well-being.

As a care team leader, you're at the heart of communication, ensuring everyone involved understands and meets your loved one's needs. It's about making decisions with clarity and compassion, advocating fiercely for your loved one's rights and preferences, and supporting your team every step of the way. You're not the solo musician anymore; now, you're the conductor, bringing together different strengths and perspectives to create a symphony of care.

Ultimately, being a care team leader ensures your loved one receives the highest quality of care possible. As a care team leader, your role involves:

1. **Finding and Equipping the Right Team:** Every family will have different needs and need other team members on board. Your job is to ensure you have the right people in the right places.

2. **Facilitating Communication**: Your role as the team leader is to ensure clear and open communication among all team members regarding your loved one's condition and care plans, and that communication flows back to you as well.

3. **Coordinating Care:** As dementia care becomes more complex, you must step into a coordination role -organizing schedules, appointments, and therapies to streamline the care process.

4. **Advocating for Your Loved One**: Even though you may be delegating certain hands-on parts of the day-to-day care to other team members, the team leader always remains the strongest advocate for the person with dementia. This means standing up for your loved one's needs, preferences, and rights throughout their care journey.

In this section, we'll discuss the essential aspects of assembling and leading a care team as a caregiver. First, we'll discuss the process of deciding how much help you need in the home. This involves assessing the specific needs of loved ones, considering factors like their medical condition, daily care requirements, and any specialized services they may require. From there, we'll address the resources available and how to find them.

Next, we'll tackle the leader's mindset and belief shifts that may be necessary as you transition into the role of a team leader. While caring for your loved one independently has challenges, coordinating a team introduces a new dynamic that requires adaptability, communication skills, and a willingness to delegate tasks effectively.

Finally, we'll cover the critical aspects of leading and managing the team. We'll start by compiling a care plan binder and then address common issues that care leaders may encounter.

By the end of this section, you'll have fully grown from a solo caregiver to a confident care leader.

Self-Reflection Questions

1. Reflect on a time when you realized you needed to expand your care team. What made you decide to hire additional help?

2. Reflect on a moment when you felt hesitant or resistant to reaching out for help expanding your care team. What were the underlying reasons for your reluctance, and how did you overcome these barriers to seek the support you needed?

Ten

Building Your Team

Dear Dr. Thomas,

My parents mean the world to me, even though we live several states apart. My father, in his late seventies, has been taking care of my mother, who has dementia, but it's become too much for him alone.

I've managed to convince my dad that bringing in help is the best way to care for Mom and protect his own health. I've spent hours researching in-home care options, reading reviews, and talking to agencies. We recently chose a small, reputable agency known for its compassionate and skilled caregivers.

I'm not sure how many hours we need to start with—the costs are high, and my parents have a fixed income right now. Do you have any advice on how to decide?

Thanks,

Jeannette

Deciding How Much Help You Need

As you step into the role of a care team leader, the first big task is forming the right team. It's about finding the perfect fit for your family's needs—too little help puts your loved one at risk, but too much can strain your finances. Like Goldilocks, it must be just right. Start by re-evaluating your loved one's needs and abilities, which we reviewed in Step 2: Lead the Care Partnership.

Here are key areas to consider:

Medical Needs: Understand any chronic conditions beyond dementia. Knowing the complexity of their medical care, including medication management needs, will help you decide if other family members can handle this or if you need specialized help.

The level of medical care needed may determine the type of help you hire. Strictly speaking, most agency caregiving aides (non-medical aides) aren't allowed to administer medications but can hand the individual their pill box. If your loved one needs someone to do more than that (like administering an insulin injection), you might need to consider hiring someone with nursing experience.

Daily Living Activities: Assess the need for assistance with personal care like bathing, dressing, and grooming, especially if mobility or cognitive issues are present. Also, consider whether help with household chores, meal preparation, and shopping is needed.

Emotional and Social Support: Consider the need for companionship and social interaction, which is crucial for mental health. Determine if there's a need for counseling or therapy to address depression, anxiety, and agitation.

Mobility and Transportation: Evaluate assistance needed for mobility and safety, including transfers and using assistive devices like walkers or wheelchairs. Also, consider if transportation help is necessary for medical visits, social outings, or errands.

Quiz: Estimating the Level of Need and Hours Needed

Instructions: Use this quiz to evaluate your loved one's needs and estimate the amount of care required. For each question, select the option that best describes the situation.

Medical Needs

- Minimal: No chronic conditions or mild, well-managed conditions (1 point)
- Moderate: One or more chronic conditions that require regular monitoring (2 points)
- High: Multiple chronic conditions requiring intensive management (3 points)

Medication Management

- No assistance needed (0 points)
- Occasional reminders (1 point)
- Daily administration and monitoring (2 points)

Personal Care

- Independent in most tasks (0 points)
- Requires help with one or two activities (1 point)
- Requires help with multiple activities (2 points)
- Completely dependent (3 points)

Household Tasks

- Independent (0 points)
- Needs help with some tasks (1 point)
- Needs help with most tasks (2 points)

Companionship

- Already has regular social interactions (0 points)
- Occasional companionship needed (1 point)
- Daily companionship needed (2 points)

Mobility Assistance

- Fully mobile (0 points)
- Needs help with mobility aids (1 point)
- Requires physical assistance (2 points)
- Bedbound (3 points)

Transportation

- Drives self or has regular transportation (0 points)
- Needs occasional transportation (1 point)
- Needs regular transportation services (2 points)

Scoring and Estimating Hours Needed: Add up the points to determine the level of need:

- **0-5 points:** Low need – Minimal care required, possibly a few hours a week up to 10 hours a week.
- **6-10 points:** Moderate need – Regular care required, potentially part-time help (10-20 hours per week).
- **11-15 points:** High need – Significant care required, likely full-time help (30-40 hours per week or more).
- **16+ points:** Very high need – Intensive care required, possibly requiring 24/7 assistance or even nursing home level of care.

The prior exercise is a general estimate based on your loved one's needs. Ultimately, you may choose to have more or less depending on your family circumstances. In addition, needs can change over time, and you may need to reassess their level of need periodically to ensure you have the right amount of help.

Types of Services Available

Please note that the quoted rates of the different services below are accurate estimates at the time of writing this book. However, they may be different based on your geographic region and market conditions. Rates quoted are in US dollars.

Now that you've assessed how *much* help your loved one needs, it's time to determine the *type* of help that will be the right fit. Remember that of the estimated hours, you are currently providing some of the caregiving support—particularly the leadership and coordination time—but you may need other types of team members to fill in the gaps.

Depending on your loved one's individual situation, you may need to consider non-medical services like companionship (mainly for social support) or home aides/personal support workers (for personal care and activities of daily living). This is the most common type of help that forms part of the care team.

Nursing care may be required if your loved one has complex medical needs. If your loved one has mobility issues, you can consider adding in-home physical, occupational, or even speech therapy to help them with swallowing, speech, and cognition. Finally, if your loved one is in the later stages or end stage of dementia, you may need the support of palliative care or hospice services to attend to their comfort needs at the end of life.

Understanding the types of services available and how to find them is crucial in building an effective care team. Each type of service can address specific needs and contribute uniquely to your loved one's well-being. In the following section of this chapter, I'll outline the different types of services you might want to consider and where you can find them.

Home Care Agencies (Non-Medical) & Private Caregivers

Home care agencies are private non-medical caregiving companies that can provide various services, from basic personal care to more specialized home support. The most common type of professional hired from a home care agency is a home health aide, sometimes called a personal support worker (PSW) or paid caregiver.

These professionals can typically be hired for personal care tasks such as bathing, dressing, medication supervision (as mentioned earlier, technically aides are not allowed to administer medications, but can hand the pillbox to your loved one), and mobility assistance. They may also assist with light housekeeping and meal preparation. Aides can be employed for as little as an hour up to 24 hours a day.

Book Portal Resource Alert!

Check your book portal for a Homecare agency interview guide.
Visit your book portal at https://www.lifecareleadhership.com/dcc

Home Care Agencies may also provide companion care, focusing on social and emotional support. Companions can help reduce feelings of loneliness and isolation by engaging the person with dementia in conversations, activities, and outings. Some companions will also help with transportation to and from appointments as long as your loved one is physically able to leave the home.

Separate from agencies, private aides and companions can also be found as independent caregivers you can contract with based on your needs – you may hear about them through word of mouth from neighbors or friends, or even through companies like care.com

Your best way to find home care agencies is through a simple Google search, as agencies vary based on geographical area. Private individuals or agencies typically charge hourly rates, which can be in the $20-$30 USD range (may vary based on your location). For 40 hours a week of care, this may look like about USD $1,000+/week in expenses.

Many agencies have minimum booking requirements, such as 3– 4-hour blocks per day, three to four times a week (i.e. 16 minimum hours per week). Private individuals through care.com or similar websites typically have more flexibility; however, you're responsible for vetting the individuals you hire.

Medicare doesn't cover private duty aides and companion services. However, long-term care insurance can be used towards this if you have it. In addition, if your loved one's income level is low, they may be eligible to have the cost of caregiving services covered through Medicaid and your local county Area Agency on Aging program (this may vary based on state regulations). Check the website of your county's Area Agency on Aging for more information.

Home Health Care Agencies (Medical)

Home Health Care Agencies offer a broad spectrum of medical services, including nursing care, physical therapy, occupational therapy, aide services, etc. Agencies will screen and train their staff, who are licensed clinicians, providing a level of assurance regarding the quality of care.

Home nurses are qualified to perform wound care, administer medication, and take care of any specialized equipment you have. They can sometimes draw lab work in the home as well. They will help you and your family learn how to care for your loved one best and teach you skills to provide home care. In addition, home nurses will report back to the physician's office if there are any medical changes to your loved one's health.

Home-based therapy includes physical therapy (which focuses on mobility), occupational therapy (which focuses on activities of daily living), and speech therapy (which focuses on speech, swallowing, and sometimes cognitive exercises). The therapists will evaluate your loved one's needs and provide recommendations for equipment and exercises to help improve their functioning.

Home health care agencies also employ home aides and may be able to send one to assist you temporarily in the home. Usually, this may cover one to two hours of home aide help per week. Some agencies will allow you to contract with them to hire an aide for additional private duty coverage.

Home Health Care agencies are covered by Medicare for a limited time, typically two to three months. A doctor's order is also required. A great place to search for these agencies is the Medicare website (https://www.medicare.gov/care-compare).

Private Duty Nursing (Medical)

Private duty nursing care is required if your loved one needs specialized medical care – like if they have tubes, drains, or a complex wound care regimen that you're unable to handle yourself.

Unfortunately, private duty nurses are difficult to find, and the cost of hiring them can be double or more than that of private duty non-medical caregivers. Depending on the situation, some insurance may cover private-duty nursing care. A Google search will be the best way to find private agencies that provide in-home nursing care.

Home Based Therapy

Home-based therapy, which includes physical, occupational, and speech-language therapy, is described in greater detail on the prior page. In some areas, you can also get in-home specialized therapy, such as therapy focused on movement disorders like Parkinson's disease or lymphedema care.

Therapy can be offered in the home through home healthcare agencies (see above) or private therapy companies.

As therapy is covered by insurance, a physician's order is required, and sometimes co-pays will apply depending on your insurance and whether you're getting it as part of home health care or separate.

Adult Day Programs

Adult day programs are typically open during working hours from Mondays to Fridays. They're not widely available, so check with the local Area Agency on Aging to find out if there's one close to you. Adult day programs may cost around $100 USD/day, but they provide meals and social activities and may provide basic healthcare and therapy needs depending on the facility. For some families, day programs are a perfect fit for their needs.

Facilities

For those requiring a higher level of care than can be provided at home, various types of facilities are available, such as assisted living, nursing homes, and memory care units. Here's a quick overview.

Assisted living facilities are apartment-style semi-independent units with a nurse in the building to help as needed. Individuals who live in assisted living facilities are typically independent of most of their care needs, but additional services– like medication management, nursing care, aide services, etc.– can be purchased as needed.

Nursing home facilities offer comprehensive care, including medical support, personal care, social activities, and 24/7 supervision. These types of facilities are needed if your loved one needs to be cared for by a nurse (for medication administration), needs more supervision, or needs one or two people for personal care and safe transfers from a bed to a wheelchair, for example.

Memory care units are an important type of facility to visit and tour, as they are staffed by nurses with dementia-specific training. Memory care units are typically locked to prevent the individual with dementia from wandering out without assistance. They fall between assisted living and nursing home levels of care.

Finding a suitable facility involves researching options, visiting potential sites, and evaluating the quality of care and environment. An excellent resource for finding facilities is the Elder Care Locator (https://eldercare.acl.gov).

Moving a loved one to an assisted living or nursing home is a bigger financial investment compared to private caregiving agencies. These facilities typically charge monthly fees covering room and board and may have extra charges for add-on services. On the plus side, you can worry less about staffing as they're required to have 24/7 coverage.

Assisted living facilities are usually structured as individual apartment units and can typically range from $4,000 to $5,000 USD per month (depending on your geographical area), plus extra for specialized care. Nursing homes range from $7,500 to $9,000 USD monthly, although this can vary based on region. Research facilities carefully to ensure they meet your loved one's needs and preferences.

Of note, neither Medicare nor Medicaid covers assisted living facilities. Long-term care at a nursing home may be covered by Medicaid or your loved one's long-term care insurance. You may need to fill out an application to see if your loved one qualifies.

Palliative Care

Palliative care is specialized medical care focused on quality of life by providing relief from the symptoms and stress of serious illness. Palliative care is suitable for anyone with an illness such as advanced heart disease, lung disease, cancer, and even dementia diagnoses. People who receive palliative care can also continue their regular doctors' appointments and pursue treatments like chemotherapy or surgery. Palliative care can be helpful for people who are in the middle, late, or end stages of dementia.

Palliative care teams often include doctors, nurses, and social workers who will work with you to improve the quality of life of your loved one with dementia.

Palliative care is covered by Medicare. They can continue receiving medical treatments, undergoing lab work, and seeing their other doctors with palliative care. Unfortunately, in-home palliative teams are not widely available, but you can check www.getpalliativecare.org to know if you can access palliative care services in your area.

Hospice Care

Hospice care is designed for individuals nearing the end of life and focuses on comfort care, pain and symptom management, and emotional support for the individual and their family. Hospice care can be provided at home or, in hospice centers, hospitals, and nursing homes. Referrals for hospice care often come from healthcare providers, as your loved one must be evaluated for hospice eligibility.

There is an unfortunate negative fear around hospice care. Many people believe that it's meant only for the last few days of life, that you have to stop all medications, and that hospice workers will come and load up your loved one with morphine, leading to their quick death. This isn't true, and in fact is the opposite of what hospice is about, however, because of this fear, most people delay hospice care until their loved one is already in the last days of their life, and they end up missing out on all of the benefits it can genuinely offer.

In reality, hospice services can be a tremendous support for the last six months (and even longer) of a person's life. Many medications are continued while on hospice care, provided that they contribute to the goals of comfort. Individuals on hospice care can be prescribed antibiotics (typically oral/tablet form) to treat minor illnesses like urinary tract infections. While morphine is prescribed to manage pain, the goal is to manage symptoms, not cause sedation.

Deciding on hospice services for your loved one can be an emotionally charged decision, and I always recommend keeping your loved ones' wishes at the forefront in the context of what's going on with their overall health. Speak with your loved one's doctor to see if hospice care is appropriate at this stage.

Hospice services are covered by Medicare, and a great place to compare hospice agencies in your area is the Medicare website (www.medicare.gov/care-compare)

In this chapter, you've made significant strides in understanding the support needed for your caregiving role. You've assessed the hours required and the types of services necessary, investigated different care options and found resources for assistance. Remember, you don't have to walk this journey alone; forming a care team can significantly benefit you and your loved one.

As you embrace your role as the care team leader, it's crucial to recognize your caregiving approach and pinpoint any gaps between what you can provide and what is required.

Self-Reflection Questions

1. After assessing the level of need and available resources mentioned in this chapter, what gaps or areas of need have you identified in your loved one's support system?

2. What type of services do you think would help bridge this gap?

Eleven

Leader's Mindset & Limiting Beliefs

Dear Dr. Thomas,

As you know, I've recently accepted that I needed help with mom and hired aides through a private agency. The first agency I used was a disaster. It seemed that these so-called professionals didn't know what they were doing. I had to show them everything, and the next day, the company sent someone else. It felt like I now had two jobs—caring for Mom and teaching their staff.

I fired them and tried a second company.

The second group was FABULOUS. I finally have the help I need and can take a break, which I sorely need.

I'm writing this email to you from my local coffee shop, which I haven't seen the inside of in years. I'm finally feeling like I'm not drowning but being the leader you always said I should be.

Diana

Perspective Shifts as You Become a Team Leader

Forming and leading a care team marks a big transition point in how you approach caring for a loved one with dementia. It's important to realize that this shift is more than just practical adjustments; it challenges deeply held beliefs about who you are and how good of a job you've done so far. Many caregivers struggle with the assumption that hiring help means they've somehow failed their job. In earlier sections of this book, we discussed how limiting beliefs can hold us back from seeing ourselves as leaders and impact our relationship with our loved ones. Overcoming these beliefs is crucial for a smooth transition to your next level up, and you do this by adopting a COO mindset – a **Leader's Mindset.**

Earlier, I shared how your role as the company's chief operating officer meant that you were responsible for running all the day-to-day operations. Until now, you've been managing it all *by doing it all*. You were the chef, the chauffeur, the janitor, and more. But now, it's time to step away from the day-to-day. As a care team leader, you need to be the one in charge of the schedule, not the one doing the day-to-day work. It would be best to shift from doing every task to overseeing and coordinating the team's efforts. This shift requires that you move from the bedside to the head of the table and take a strategic approach to ensure your loved one receives comprehensive care. Recognizing and embracing this Leader's Mindset shift is critical to successfully leading a care team.

In this chapter, we'll study three key perspective shifts:

- "It's easier to do this solo than to train others."
- "I have to double-check everything to ensure it's done right."
- "Having a team is an expensive cost I can't afford."

Now, let's explore these beliefs and how they might affect your ability to lead a care team effectively.

Perspective Shift#1: "It's Easier to do This Solo Than Have to Train Others" to..."Training Someone Takes Time and Effort, But It Is Worth the Effort"

The first perspective shift centers around the mindset changes that occur when you go from solo caregiving to employing your team. Even the first hire, the first helper, can feel daunting, much like Diana expressed in her letter earlier.

You may find it hard to trust others with tasks and prefer handling everything yourself. Training someone new often takes considerable time and effort. There's also the risk that it might not work out despite your best efforts, or they quit and you have to start all over again. This cycle can be discouraging and make you wonder why you even bothered.

However, continuing to handle everything alone can lead to burnout, as your loved one's needs will continue to grow. As their care requirements increase, so does your daily workload, which may become unsustainable without support. Introducing a team early allows your loved one to adjust and build trust with new caregivers. This transition period is crucial for them to feel comfortable and lessen their dependence solely on you.

To help you shift from solo to team, try the exercise on the next page to practice documenting a workflow, process, or task for a new team member.

Exercise: Documenting Processes and Delegating Tasks

1. **Identify the Task:** Choose a caregiving task you find takes up a lot of your time or effort.

2. **Identify Expectations:** Identify the good/better/best goals for this task. What does acceptable look like?

3. **Create a Step-By-Step Instruction Guide:** Next, write down exactly how you would want your team member to do the process, starting at the very beginning. Imagine you're watching yourself doing the tasks on a video and identify each part of the process, breaking it down into basic steps. Write them all down.

4. **Set a Goal:** Discuss the caregiving plan and instruction guide with your team member today. Don't expect perfection on day; you may still need to demonstrate what and how you want them to do things. However, you now have clear expectations and instructions that they can refer to when needed.

Remember, when you start looking for additional help in caregiving, you won't find the perfect person on your first try. You might need to interview and try a few different agencies before finding the right fit. Training someone to care for your loved one the way you expect takes time and effort, but the effort is worth it. The purpose of building a care team is ultimately to reduce burnout *while* ensuring your loved one receives the best possible care.

Perspective shift #2: "I Have to Double-Check Everything Done to Make Sure It's Done Right." to… "I Will Train Them Well the First Time and Then Supervise and Intervene Only When Needed."

Perfectionism can be a tough habit to break, especially when working with a caregiving team, as we've encountered in other chapters. In leading a team, perfectionism can look like micromanaging.

> *Joann's Story:* Joann had been the primary caregiver for her husband for years before she decided to hire private aides from a caregiving agency. Joann's most significant challenge was stopping herself from constantly intervening and criticizing the caregivers' methods. She would get upset when things weren't done exactly her way, redoing the work that had already been done. This led to arguments, and eventually the caregiver quit on a weekend when Joann especially needed help.

It's important to remember that if you're not happy with the help you're getting, it's your responsibility as the team leader to address it. Sometimes, this means having a constructive talk with the caregiver; other times, it means taking your concerns to their supervisor or requesting a different caregiver. You're paying for these services, so you should feel comfortable with the people in your home.

However, there's a big difference between supervision and micromanagement. If you're constantly critiquing, double-checking, and redoing your assigned work, you're not leading effectively. It means you don't trust the people you've hired or that they're not skilled enough (meaning you should hire someone else).

Like I said earlier, leading a team means taking a step back, and if you're constantly in the trenches doing and redoing the day-to-day caregiving tasks, you're not *leading*. Experienced caregivers in particular might feel undervalued if their skills and experience aren't trusted, and they will leave. Like any other job, no one likes working for a boss who doesn't trust them.

Exercise: Lead, Don't Micromanage

1. **Set Clear Expectations:** Expectations should be communicated clearly with caregivers at the start of their time with you.

2. **Observe Objectively**: Now it's time to step back and observe how they do. When caregivers go above and beyond, make sure you acknowledge their efforts.

3. **Build Trust:** Practice letting go of small mistakes and focus on the bigger picture. Trust your caregivers to handle tasks their way, if the outcome meets your standards.

4. **If Standards are Not Met**: if you've been clear on expectations, provided clear instructions and even had the grace to let go of small mistakes, but if the caregiver is still unable to meet your acceptable standards, it's time to let them go.

By using the steps above, you'll approach your loved one's caregiving needs and team members' performance from the perspective of a leader. Remember, your goal should be to hire and train well so that you can step back and let them do the work they're assigned to do.

Perspective Shift#3: "Having a Team Is an Expensive Cost I Cannot Afford" to…"Having a Good Team Is a Worthwhile Investment"

The third perspective shift concerns expense, money, and cost. Many caregivers see hiring help as a cost rather than an investment. Remember, you're either paying with your own energy and time, or you're paying with cash for someone else's help. Let's learn how Cara realized the value of paying for in-home help.

> *Cara's story*: Cara was afraid to hire help because she worried about her long-term financial security. At the same time, she couldn't manage her husband's care needs alone, but kept putting off hiring a caregiver. Unfortunately, her husband suffered a fall that resulted in a hip fracture. He then needed to be placed in a nursing home, which ended up being much costlier than in-home help before the fall.

Realizing that paying for additional help isn't a small amount of money can be daunting, especially when you're already dealing with financial constraints and fixed incomes. It often feels like an expense beyond what you can afford. This worry is understandable, given how it can impact your finances immediately. However, it's important to reframe this mindset and think about the long-term benefits of investing in the right kind of support.

The cost of professional caregiving services might seem very high, and many families immediately feel the financial strain. However, consider the alternative—nursing home placement, which often comes with even higher ongoing expenses. Investing in the correct type of support, even in small amounts early on, might avoid or delay the high financial costs of nursing home placement. Plus, there are invaluable benefits: your loved one's well-being, their safety, and your peace of mind.

Exercise: Asset vs. Liability?

1. **List the Costs:** Write down the costs of in-home care versus nursing home care. Compare the immediate and long-term expenses. (If you aren't sure of what to expect, I've outlined some of the cost ranges in the last chapter)

2. **Think Long-Term:** Consider the potential savings of preventing accidents and hospital stays by having in-home care.

3. **Value Peace of Mind:** Reflect on the non-financial benefits, like knowing your loved one is safe and well-cared for at home. On the other side, there's a new stress that's added – making sure the paid caregivers arrive on time and are available when you need it

4. **Assess Financial Resources:** Look into what financial resources your loved one has. Do they have assets, retirement savings, life insurance, or disability insurance that can help cover caregiving costs?

5. **Explore Additional Resources:** Through the local county, Area Agency on Aging, and Medicaid, families are sometimes able to get the costs of caregivers covered. This will be based on your loved one's income level, and you'll need to check and see if you qualify.

By shifting your perspective and seeing in-home care as a valuable investment, you can make decisions that benefit your loved one and your financial future.

Embracing the Mindset of a Care Leader

As a care leader, you should no longer be immersed in the daily tasks but sit at the head of the table, thinking strategically, planning for the long term, and finding the right people to join your team.

Understanding and planning for long-term needs is key to being a care leader. This might involve assessing future care needs when dementia progresses, and making sure there is a sustainable and financially sound care plan in place. By thinking long-term, you can make better decisions that will benefit your loved one over time.

As a care leader, you understand that not just anyone can do the job. Finding the right people is crucial. You want team members who are skilled, trustworthy, and compassionate. Your team should complement each other's strengths and provide the best care for your loved one. It's about building a team you can rely on and who genuinely cares about your loved one's well-being.

Everything changes when you start seeing your team as an asset rather than a cost. Each member brings unique skills and perspectives that enhance the quality of care. Investing in your team pays off in the long run. A strong and reliable team can significantly improve the care your loved one receives and reduce your stress and workload.

Here at the end of this chapter, you have learned the importance of shifting your perspective from being the sole person responsible for care to becoming a care team leader. In the next chapter, we'll help you learn how to connect with and manage your team.

Self-Reflection Questions

1. Is it worth investing the time to train others, even if it's challenging in the beginning?

2. How can reframing caregiving expenses as a strategic investment help you accept and hire helpers?

Twelve

Team Coordination & Management

Dear Dr. Thomas,

I wanted to share how much I've grown on this caregiving journey with Mark.

When Mark was diagnosed with Alzheimer's dementia, I managed his meds, helped with daily tasks, and supported him emotionally every day. But as Mark's condition got worse, I started feeling overwhelmed and tired.

I knew I had to change things to give Mark the best care possible. So, I decided to become a care team leader, like you've always advised me. I reached out for help and built a strong support system around us.

Nowadays, I confidently manage Mark's care and take better care of myself. Thank you for your support and advice over the years. I look forward to continuing to learn from you on this journey.

Elizabeth

Connecting with Your Team

We're now in the last step of the Confident Care Leader Framework, Step 3: Leading the Care Team. In the prior chapters of this step, you identified your team and overcame the mindset blocks that were holding you back.

In this chapter, I want you to remember the importance of connecting with your team. This connection is what differentiates good leaders from the best leaders. The team that you've assembled—whether they are family members or paid private duty staff—is your team. When you see them as *your* team, their success becomes your success.

Communication is, of course, the foundation of all connections as a team leader. As the team leader, you want to make sure that information flows clearly between you, the rest of the team, and any external (out-of-home) teams like doctors' offices.

Communication is just the first step, however. When you connect with your team members on a deeper level, you find common ground, respect the individual who's there with you, and learn to hold each other accountable—you as the leader and them as the team member. The deeper the connection with your team, the higher the return on your investment—people want to work with a leader who genuinely cares for them, and they'll put in their best effort as a result.

As a care team leader, look for ways to find common ground with your team. The apparent commonality will be your shared objective: the health, safety, and happiness of your loved one with dementia. There may be other things you have in common, and the more connections you build, the stronger the team relationship will be.

Respecting the individual means understanding they're human beings with their own responsibilities and lives, but that they're also professionals hired for a purpose. Being clear and upfront on expectations is one way of being respectful and accountable to each other.

As the team leader, you're also accountable to your team – if their success is your success, then you want to make sure they have the necessary information, tools, and environment to do their job well. One tool I always recommend is a centralized document or binder that contains the care plan.

Creating a Care Plan Document

A care plan isn't just paperwork—it's a dynamic guide that shapes the support your loved one receives. This living and evolving document should outline their daily routines, medical needs, and emotional support requirements. It ensures that everyone involved—caregivers, family, and friends—understands their roles, the timing of tasks, and their responsibilities in providing consistent care.

Preparing a care plan starts by transforming your understanding of your loved one's needs, gathered in prior sections of this book, into a structured framework that clarifies who will do what, when, and how. It's a communication book that ensures everyone's the same page. In the last chapter, you identified the individuals who will be your care team—professional caregivers and family and friends' support. Now it's time to synthesize all this information into a cohesive roadmap for care.

You must organize all this information and resources in a secure and accessible format, such as a binder, or you could use an expanding file folder. This will make it easy to change or update sections as needed. You can customize your binder in whatever way makes most sense for your needs, but here are a few things you'll always want to include:

- **Emergency Information**: Ensure you have emergency contact numbers, including family members, neighbors, and the primary care physician. This information should also be placed in a visible spot – like on the refrigerator.

- **Medical Problem List**: List important diagnoses, conditions, and surgeries with dates.

- **Medication List:** Maintain an up-to-date list of all medications, dosages, frequencies, and special instructions. This list must be checked frequently for accuracy, and a copy must always be brought to any doctor's appointments.

- **Allergies**: Document any known allergies, including specific reactions and any emergency response procedures – like how to administer an Epi-Pen if they have one.

- **Doctors' Office Numbers:** Keep a list of all healthcare providers involved in your loved one's care, along with their specialties and contact information.

- **Advanced Care Planning Records**: Include any advanced care directives, living wills, or other legal documents related to end-of-life care preferences and medical power of attorney.

Additionally, you may want to include:

- **Team Communication Notes**: Use the binder as a central storage space for team communication, where everyone can document updates or changes to your loved one's condition while under your care.
- **Care Team Members & Responsibilities:** List all members of the care team, including their roles, responsibilities, and contact information.
- **Contact Information for Agencies:** Include contact details for agencies or organizations involved in your loved one's care, such as home care agencies or hospice services.
- **Your Instruction Guide**: If you have specific instructions and expectations for tasks, include them here.
- **Contracts**: If applicable, include copies of contracts or agreements with caregivers, agencies, or other service providers.
- **Medical Equipment Providers**: If your loved one has medical equipment like a hospital bed or a wheelchair, list the name and contact information for any durable medical equipment companies so that you can easily contact them in case of servicing needs.
- **Symptom Log:** Track changes in symptoms or behaviors, noting their frequency and severity and if any changes occur. For example, bowel movement frequency should be tracked for individuals with constipation issues.
- **Routines**: Document daily schedules, including mealtimes, medication schedules, appointments, and recreational activities, to provide stability and reduce anxiety.

- **Likes and Dislikes**: Record your loved one's preferences, such as favorite foods, activities, hobbies, and music, to enhance their quality of life. This can be helpful for caregivers who are new to your loved one.

Remember, a care plan isn't just a piece of paper but a central hub for organizing and coordinating all aspects of your loved one's care. This binder will evolve, reflecting changes in your loved one's condition.

> ***Book Portal Resource Alert!***
> Look for sample care plan templates in your book portal.
> Visit your book portal at https://www.lifecareleadhership.com/dcc

Implementing the Care Plan

Executing the care plan involves turning your well-thought-out strategy into daily actions that enhance your loved one's quality of life.

As the leader of the care team, your role is pivotal. You'll coordinate schedules, communicate with team members, monitor progress, and adjust as needed. This process demands flexibility, adaptability, and clear communication among all involved.

Each care team member plays a vital role in executing the plan effectively. Whether administering medication, assisting with personal care, providing companionship, or managing household tasks, every task contributes significantly to your loved one's overall well-being. It's essential to clearly assign responsibilities in your care plan and communicate expectations effectively with each team member.

Executing the care plan also requires ongoing evaluation and refinement. As you implement the plan, you'll assess what works well and what needs improvement. Gathering feedback from team members and monitoring your loved one's response to the care provided will guide adjustments to ensure the plan remains effective and adaptable to your loved one's evolving needs.

Specific Challenges when Leading the Care Team

This section has discussed several changes that you, as a caregiver, need to embrace as you become the team leader. But as anyone who's had to lead a team of any size knows, the larger the group, the more complexity and room for challenging interactions. We'll address a few of these challenges you might encounter when leading the care team for your loved one.

#1: Challenging Family Dynamics

The stress of caring for an ill or aging loved one can magnify differences in opinions, priorities, and past issues. Illnesses like dementia are stressful for everyone involved, and as the care team leader, it may be hard to keep everyone on the same page and in alignment with your overall vision. It's common for family members who were previously uninvolved to show up out of the blue, making demands for changes, but then not stay to implement the actions themselves.

Ideally, the person providing the majority of the care and care leadership – you – is also the one with the authority to make medical and financial decisions to implement the care plan. However, this isn't the case in many family situations; sometimes, a different family member is the POA (power of attorney) agent. In other family scenarios, no one has explicitly been appointed, and the primary caregiver may need to make decisions for the rest of the family first. Whatever your family scenario is, here are some tips to streamline the process:

Action Steps: Challenging Family Dynamics

1. **Schedule Regular Family Meetings**: Plan regular meetings or discussions to provide a structured platform for family members to express concerns, share viewpoints, and work together on caregiving decisions.
2. **Establish Ground Rules for Communication**: Set up guidelines that encourage respectful and constructive conversations during family meet-

ings. Stress the importance of discussing issues calmly and objectively to prevent conflicts from escalating.

3. **Identify and Address Concerns:** Encourage family members to openly share their worries and r cognize that disagreements are normal under stressful circumstances. Look for common ground and potential compromises that prioritize your loved one's well-being.
4. **Clarify Roles and Responsibilities:** Define and clarify the roles of each family member within the care team. Appreciate that each person is bringing a unique contribution to caregiving.
5. **Seek Mediation or Professional Guidance:** If conflicts persist or become difficult to resolve, consider seeking mediation or guidance from a counselor who specializes in family dynamics.

#2: Team Member Performance & Accountability Issues

Another common issue that caregivers of a loved one with dementia face is what to do when a member of the team, such as a private paid caregiver, fails to meet expectations. For instance, consider a scenario where an aide in sick repeatedly, is a no-show for their appointed shift, or spends most of their time on their phone when they're supposed to be caring for your loved one.

There are two skills you need to develop to handle these types of situations: (1) setting expectations and then (2) holding the team accountable to the expectations. We talked in prior chapters about the importance of setting expectations and using the Good/Better/Best framework to create standards you expect. This also applies to things like timeliness and reporting callouts or absences. As the team leader, you must know if the team will be there when needed.

It's important that you lay out these expectations upfront so there's no question about what was required. Remember, we're aiming for acceptable, so we expect a basic level of professionalism from other team members. The next step is holding the team accountable for meeting these expectations, especially if they're unmet. Here are some steps you should follow, using caregiver tardiness as an example.

Action Steps: Team Member Accountability – Lateness

1. **Document the Issue**: Keep a record of instances where lateness affects the care schedule.
2. **Three Strikes – Time to Discuss**: Schedule a one-on-one talk to address the issue.
3. **Listen First:** Naturally, the team member will have reasons for why they were unable to meet the expectation. Some reasons may have been out of their control, acknowledge that the caregiver is a human being too, and that they're trying their best.
4. **Once again clarify expectations, and outline consequences:** Be clear on the expectations and outline the consequence of repeat tardiness. They may be fired immediately, it may escalate to their boss, or some other consequence.
5. **Follow Up**: After addressing the issue, follow up with the team member to make sure expectations continue to be met. If they aren't, you need to follow through on the consequences you outlined previously.

#3: Navigating the Challenges of the Healthcare System

As a physician, I know how broken the system can be, especially for family caregivers struggling to get answers to sometimes basic questions. In today's modern medicine, getting more than ten minutes' time with the doctor is hard, and appointments may need to be booked months in advance. When you need help at the moment, it's hard to find.

The other healthcare-related issue that many caregivers face is conflicting information. Often, one specialist will prescribe a medication or a treatment plan that conflicts entirely with the other doctor's plans. It feels like no one is talking to each other. Medication errors happen far too often for older adults because of the communication breakdowns between healthcare and caregiving teams. In the end, it's the person with dementia who suffers.

Unfortunately, I don't have a good solution to the problems facing healthcare as a whole. Still, I know that many older adults would suffer tremendously without care leaders like yourself advocating for your loved ones.

Here are a few tips for interacting with the health system to get the most out of your appointments.

Action Steps: Working with the Healthcare System

1. **Keep your own copies of medical records in both print and digital versions.**

2. **Prepare for Appointments**: Write down your questions and concerns ahead of time, and bring a list of all medications, including over-the-counter drugs and supplements. This preparation can help make the most of the limited time you have with the doctor.

3. **Use technology to your advantage**: Many healthcare providers offer patient portals where you can access medical records, communicate with doctors, and manage appointments. Utilize these tools to stay informed and involved in your loved one's care. Note that complex questions should be reserved for in-person visits.

4. **Stay Organized**: Keep a dedicated notebook or digital file for notes from appointments, questions, and any changes in your loved one's condition. This can help you track progress and communicate effectively with healthcare providers.

5. **Utilize Care Navigators, Social Workers and Support Groups:** Care navigators are often nurses or social workers who work independently or in partnership with your doctor's office to help with coordination of care. Ask your primary care doctor's office if they can recommend you to a care navigator in your region. Also, ask for referrals to local dementia care support groups that may be hosted by the nearby hospital system.

Stepping into the role of care team leader is the start of your journey. Along the way, you might sometimes feel unsure or frustrated—it's natural. But remember, leading isn't supposed to feel easy; it requires stretching yourself. Only through this growth will you become the leader your loved one needs. You can make a real difference with a supportive team and a shared goal of caring for your loved one.

Self-Reflection Questions

1. Think about a recent interaction you had with the healthcare system. What steps can you take to better prepare for future appointments and ensure clear communication with your loved one's doctors?
2. Review your current care plan and support system. Identify one area where you can immediately improve to enhance coordination and ensure everyone understands their roles and responsibilities.

Step 3 Recap

Lead the Care Team

As we conclude our journey into care leadership through this third step, let's reflect on the transformative growth you've experienced so far:

Why You Need a Team

In the first chapter of this section, we highlighted the importance of having a team, and your specific roles and responsibilities as the team leader.

Building Your Team

In this chapter, we identified who should be on your team and how much help you need based on your loved one's current needs and abilities. We also reviewed different types of services and where to find them.

Leader's Mindset & Limiting Beliefs as Team Leader

Next, we discussed the essential perspective shifts required as you transition into a care team leader. Going from solo caregiver to managing a team can be a big step and may require a big change in perspective.

Team Coordination & Management

Lastly, we explored how you can effectively manage your team for success. It starts with compiling a care plan binder containing all the details you've worked so hard to put together in this book. Writing a plan isn't enough, though, because executing it requires your oversight and coordination. In this last chapter of this section, we reviewed everyday struggles that care leaders experience with their teams and how to work through them.

Let's turn the page to the book's closing section and ensure your long-term success!

ENSURING YOUR LONG TERM SUCCESS

Caregiving often calls us to lean into love we didn't know possible.

Tia Walker

Dear Reader,

Congratulations on making it this far in your care leadership journey!

As a family caregiver for a loved one with dementia, you've shown incredible strength to get to the last few pages of this book. While you may feel like you've reached the end, you're actually just beginning to unlock your potential as a care team leader.

Now it's time to look back and see how much you've grown. Do you remember the self-assessment quiz we did in the introduction to this book? Let's repeat the quiz now and see how far you've come by comparing it to your results from Chapter 1.

Care Leader Self-Assessment:

Instructions: Rate your confidence level on a scale from 1 to 10, where 1 = Not Confident and 10 = Very Confident.

1. ________My confidence in understanding and utilizing my unique skills as a care leader.

2. ________My confidence in creating and maintaining a wellness plan for my own well-being.

3. ________My confidence in accurately assessing and understanding the needs of my loved one.

4. ________My confidence in communicating with my loved one to ensure their needs and preferences are met.

5. ________My confidence in identifying the right people to include in my care team

6. ________My confidence in creating a care plan that enables all team members to work together effectively

As you continue to grow and evolve as a care leader, remember that it's normal to experience ups and downs. There will always be new things to learn, and while this book has a lot of resources, it's just the starting place for your individual growth. Perhaps you need to focus more on communication, team management, or even your own self-care. The more you grow, the stronger the team leader you'll become.

One of the most important factors in ensuring your long-term success as a care leader is surrounding yourself with a supportive community of fellow caregivers who understand your journey. This community can provide invaluable support, guidance, and encouragement.

Community support can come in many forms, from local caregiver support groups to online forums and social media communities. Connecting with other caregivers allows you to share experiences, learn from each other's successes and challenges, and find solidarity, knowing you're not alone on this journey.

Additionally, consider seeking out more structured forms of support, such as caregiver coaching programs or courses specifically tailored to caregivers of loved ones with dementia. These programs can provide personalized guidance, practical skills, and emotional support to help you thrive as a care leader.

As a palliative care physician and a caregiving coach, I've witnessed firsthand the transformative power of coaching. Women like you, who may have once felt overwhelmed and burnt out, have emerged confident, empowered leaders.

By embracing their role as care leaders, these women have learned to delegate tasks, set boundaries, and prioritize their well-being without sacrificing the quality of care for their loved ones. They've cultivated strong support networks within their families and communities and found fulfillment in knowing they're making a positive difference in their loved ones' lives.

As a result of their growth and transformation, they and their loved ones enjoy happier, healthier, and more fulfilling lives. They've learned that being a care leader is not just about managing tasks and responsibilities; it's about leading with compassion, resilience, and grace.

Now that you're done with this book, I invite you to join me in one of my courses or coaching programs, designed specifically for female caregivers of loved ones with dementia just like you.

Through these programs and courses, you'll have the opportunity to further develop and strengthen the leadership skills we've learned together in this book while being a part of a supportive community.

As you continue your caregiving journey, remember to lead with heart and care with purpose.

Your friend,

Dr. Anna Thomas

www.lifecareleadership.com

I look forward to seeing you there!

About The Author

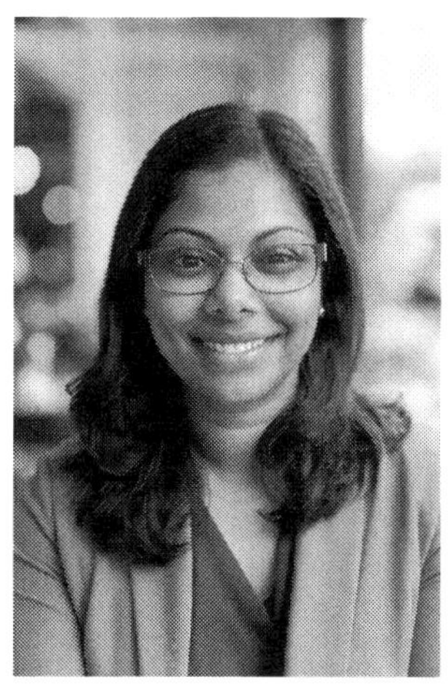

Dr. Anna Thomas is a board-certified internist and hospice and palliative care physician who dedicated her career to supporting individuals through life's most challenging moments.

Her personal experiences within her own family have profoundly shaped her journey in dementia care. Driven by these insights and work experiences, she has made it her mission to empower female caregivers.

She is the founder of LifeCare LeadHership, a coaching company focused solely on the needs of female caregivers. Through LifeCare LeadHership, she provides personalized coaching, education, and training to support female caregivers as they navigate the challenges of dementia care.

Dr. Thomas believes that all caregivers are care leaders and can lead with heart and care with purpose by unlocking their inner leadership strengths.

You can learn more about Dr. Thomas at her website:
https://www.lifecareleadhership.com

Made in the USA
Middletown, DE
01 November 2024

63226594R00088